Also by Cynthia Stamper Graff:

Lean for Life Phase One: Weight Loss
(with Jerry Holderman)

bodyPRIDE
(with Janet Eastman & Mark C. Smith)

Lean for Life ®

PHASE TWO
LIFETIME SOLUTIONS

SECOND EDITION

CYNTHIA STAMPER GRAFF

Foreward by
JOHN P. FOREYT, Ph.D.
Director, Behavioral Medicine Research Center
Baylor College of Medicine
Houston, Texas

Griffin Publishing Group

Griffin Publishing Group
18022 Cowan, Suite 202
Irvine, California 92614

Library of Congress Cataloging-in-Publication Data

Graff, Cynthia Stamper
Lean for Life Phase Two: Lifetime Solutions /by Cynthia Stamper Graff.

1. Weight Maintenance. 2. Diet. 3. Weight Loss. 4. Health.
5. Fitness 6. Nutrition. I. Title.

ISBN 1-58000-089-4

Second Edition
Printed in the United States of America

10 9 8 7 6 5 4

Lean for Life® and Mitrochrondriac® are registered trademarks of Lindora, Inc., Costa Mesa, California.

This book is dedicated to
all those who have struggled
to maintain their weight,
and have refused to give in or give up.

Tell me... I'll forget.
Show me... I'll remember.
Involve me... I'll understand.

TABLE OF CONTENTS

WEEK 1
BALANCE: THE ART OF MAINTENANCE

Losing and Maintaining: As So It Goes
EAT BETTER: Your Daily Action Plan
MOVE MORE: What Successful Maintainers Say About Exercise
STRESS LESS: Laughing Yourself Well
Success Story: Carol Consolo

A Worthy Goal
EAT BETTER: All Foods Are Not Created Equal
MOVE MORE: Following Your Tracks
STRESS LESS: When You're Smiling, the Whole World Smiles with You
MENTAL FITNESS: The Scale is Your Friend
What is Your BMI?

Maintaining Small Losses Equals Big Health Gains
EAT BETTER: What Should I Eat?
MOVE MORE: Moderate but Steady Always Wins the Race
STRESS LESS: The Basics of Relaxation
Brain Food: The National Weight Control Registry

WEEK 2
INTENTION: THE CAPACITY TO ACT CONSCIOUSLY

WEEK 3
THE STRATEGY OF BALANCED EATING

WEEK 4
MOVEMENT: THE BEAUTY OF A WELL-USED BODY

MOVE MORE: Resistance Training
STRESS LESS: A Letter of Appreciation
Binge Eating Disorder

A Well-Used Body
EAT BETTER: Help for Binge-Eaters
MOVE MORE: Yoga Breathing
STRESS LESS: Loving through Listening
MENTAL FITNESS: Visualizing the Journey

Seeing with Different Eyes
EAT BETTER: Protein
MOVE MORE: Exercise and Addictions
STRESS LESS: Depression
How Do You Feel About Your Body?

WEEK 5
PROBLEM-SOLVING: THE ABILITY TO FIGURE IT OUT

Keeping At It
EAT BETTER: Feeling Full
MOVE MORE: Maintaining Your Fitness Gains
STRESS LESS: Giving It a Name
MENTAL FITNESS: What Makes People Stick to It?

Reading the Signals
EAT BETTER: The Paleolithic Diet
MOVE MORE: How Walking Combats the Common Cold
STRESS LESS: The Three-Minute Time Out
MENTAL FITNESS: A Meditation for Perspective

An Objective Look
EAT BETTER: Cutting Back After You've Overindulged
MOVE MORE: Increasing Your Activity After You've Overindulged
STRESS LESS: Loving Yourself Anyway
Success Story: Ivy Williams

WEEK 6
MENTAL STRENGTH: THE KEY TO CHANGE

WEEK 7
HUMAN CONNECTION: THE ESSENCE OF HEALTH

WEEK 8
COMMITMENT: THE ENERGY TO KEEP GOING

MOVE MORE: Second Wind
STRESS LESS: Letting a Child Choose
MENTAL FITNESS: More on Creativity

Flying Solo
EAT BETTER: New Recipes
MOVE MORE: One Last Plea for Keeping Track
STRESS LESS: A Simple Gift

Congratulations!
Success Story: Sandra Radine

SPECIAL APPRECIATION

I want to express my gratitude and special appreciation to two gifted people whose efforts, energy, and extraordinary commitment to excellence have made working on this book a true pleasure:

Jean Coppock Staeheli

Jean Coppock Staeheli's remarkable gift of words and spirit are evident on every page of this book. She is a rare and wonderful human being who, through her great wisdom and personal energy, definitely brings out the very best I have within me. Her focus, clarity of thought, and quiet strength are a true inspiration. It was an honor to collaborate with Jean on this book.

Jerry Holderman

Jerry Holderman possesses a unique blend of creative talent, strong organizational skills, and a truly collaborative spirit, all of which were well-utilized in the development of this book. His feature profiles of the inspiring people whose "Success Stories" appear throughout this book give it a valuable added dimension. With his fine eye for design, keen attention to detail and deadlines, and his very special way with words, Jerry contributed significantly to the book you are holding.

ACKNOWLEDGMENTS

This book would not exist if it weren't for the genius of my father, Marshall B. Stamper, M.D. As a clinician in the field of obesity treatment, he is truly in a class with few equals. I have been the fortunate recipient of his vast knowledge base, partially through osmosis (just being around him over many years), partially through genetic predisposition (which I think must explain the passion I feel for the work we do), but mostly because he cared enough about his patients to want to share all he had learned from his experiences with them.

While the intellectual inspiration for this book belongs to my father, the heart that is woven throughout is inspired by my mother, Nell Stamper, and reinforced by my terrific brothers, Steve Stamper and Bernie Stamper, and my wonderful sister, Kitty Nordstrom. I am blessed to be part of the Stamper family.

This book is a collaborative effort with input and support from many sources and many special people. The energy, wisdom, love, and commitment from a remarkable team of people has helped create a finished product that feels greater than the sum of its parts.

First, I want to thank the many Lindora patients who share their struggles and successes with us day in and day out. We hear remarkable success stories nearly every day, and we're pleased to be able to share some of them in this book. Special thanks to Jason Andrews, Barbra Bercarich, Carol Consolo, Theresa Davis, Richard Evanns, Mark Huckenpahler, Austin Kovac, Sonya LaRusso, Dr. Tari Lennon, John Morgan, Sandra Radine, Tammy Randall, Donna Smith, and Ivy Williams for allowing us to share their stories in this book.

There aren't enough positive adjectives to describe the physicians, nurses, nurse practitioners, clinic and administrative team members of Lindora. Through their dedication to excellence and their compassionate treatment of our patients, they have created the largest clinical organization in America specializing in the treatment of overweight and obesity. Special thanks to Laura Kanuk, Katherine Trueblood, Sandy DeLella, Peggy Dewitt, R.N., Shirley Prather, L.V.N., Pam Bage, Jayme Davidson, R.N., Jodi Kinzel, R.N., Carol Mulvey, L.V.N., Cynthia Powers, R.N., Kathy Walker, R.N., Jackie Martinez, L.V.N., Terry Chronister, L.V.N., and Vickie Flatt, L.V.N. for their help in referring the people whose "Success Stories" we've shared in this book.

Debbie Riley, L.V.N., Lindora's Nurse Educator, once again came through her usual insight and dedication.

Joseph Risser, M.D., M.P.H., our director of Clinical Research, deserves a hug for the time he spent researching for me, reviewing the manuscript, as well as actually treating Lindora patients, thereby contributing to our rapidly expanding data base of knowledge and experience.

Thank you to Andral Dugger, M.D., Judi Goldstone, M.D., John Dubois, M.D., Lynne Nieto, N.P., Cay Taylor, N.P., Jeanette Schmidt, N.P., and Patricia O'Donnell, N.P., for their dedication and exceptional patient care; special thanks to Lynne Nieto for developing training materials based on this book.

I want to express my sincere appreciation for my entire administrative team. Their commitment to the Lindora mission makes it possible for our clinical staff to concentrate on exceptional patient care and know their operational needs will be met. Thank you to Jeff Beltz, Leon Lombardo, Todd Cornish, Danielle Gray, Al Andres, Vince Duong, John Hendricks, James Scott, Adam Chan, Melanie Dingle, Rauha Hilander, Kristina Gerke, Dalonda Mahony, Gustavo Rivera, Thao Tran, Christine Gil, Joseph Walton, Michelle Wikle, Mike Quinn, Patti Sewell, Albert Smith, Karen TerBorg, Mike Kollen, Corinne Wikle, Mark Wisniewski, and Pam Withers. I greatly appreciate the "can do" attitude of Keith McGuinness, Stella Gates, Sherrie Theckston, Ryan Mariden, and Donna Rockenbach.

Thanks to Leslie Wulff, R.N., our Vice President of Clinical Operations, for her inspiring leadership.

Thanks to Olivia Beltz, Stacie Yee, and Georgia Zachariah for all you do to make my job—and my life—easier.

To my assistant, Billye Shinto Littman: you help me in more ways than you know with your creativity and insight. Thank you.

I'm grateful for the wise counsel of Roger Riddell. Chris Keenan deserves acknowledgment for constantly bringing us new ideas. Karen York, a kindred spirit, has contributed so much to our enterprise and thus to this book.

A sincere thanks to Peter Vash, M.D., M.P.H., our wonderful Executive Medical Director. His contributions in the field of Bariatric medicine are noteworthy, and his dedication and contributions to Lindora over the years has garnered both respect and admiration. Thank you, Peter.

I would also like to acknowledge the commited associates of HealthNet in California, a part of Foundation Health Systems. They deserve the reputation they've earned for being a leader among the managed care organizations in the field of preventive medicine. Lindora is proud to be one of their WellRewards partners. This book is, in part, a response to a request from a Health Net member for a structured long-term maintenance program. I greatly appreciate the confidence in our program that Blue Cross of California and UNICARE have demonstrated by making Lean for Life available to their members.

Ellen McGrath, Ph.D., a most gifted psychologist, has shown me that it does indeed take a village to raise an adult. Her wisdom regarding the need for human "connection" is reflected in many places throughout this book.

Thanks to Harry Wexler, Ph.D., and Pia Santiago for their innovative research on the association between obesity and depression among Lindora patients. We always knew that our patients seemed healthier and happier when they maintained active contact with us, and we now have the tools and research to validate those clinical observations.

The terms for two of the main strategies featured in this book come from an exemplary community program called "Sisters Together" in Boston, Massachusetts. I was so taken with the simple elegance of their logo, "Eat Better, Move More". These words sum up a copious and complex amount of material on this subject in a way that is easily and readily understood.

I want to thank Lance Huante and his team at p11 creative. Their creative clarity has contributed greatly to the look and feel of this book, and I appreciate their talents. Thanks to Elizabeth Hargreaves and her team at Pure Octane, and to Bob Hodson. Thanks, too, to Frank Groff for his unstoppable energy, to Herman M. Frankel, M.D. for his ongoing support in my own mental training and personal growth, and to the team at Griffin Publishing Group for their continuing belief in our programs and the value of getting them out into the world.

There are several giants in the field of obesity research who have impacted and influenced the program presented in this book. I am privileged to have been present at lectures given by the Senior Statesman of the field, Albert Stunkard, M.D.. I continue to be inspired by George Blackburn, M.D., Ph.D. as well as the stellar group of leading experts who make presentations at the annual Harvard Obesity Conference: Steven Blair, P.E.D., Barbara Corkey, Ph.D., Judy Stern, Ph.D., Rena Wing, Ph.D., Xavier Pi-Sunyer, M.D., M.P.H., Susan Yanovski, M.D., Richard Atkinson, M.D., William Dietz, M.D., Kelly Brownell, Ph.D., and Thomas Wadden, Ph.D., who has been especially helpful with his keen insights.

I appreciate the support that is given to the field by two fine organizations. First, the North American Society of Obesity (NASSO). It was an honor to accompany Dr. Peter Vash to the International Obesity Conference in Paris, where he presented data based on long-term Lindora patient outcomes. Thank you, too, to the American Society of Bariatric Physicians for their educational support. Special thanks to Jim Merker, C.A.E., and his staff, and to Larry Richardson, M.D.

Last but certainly not least, I owe a special debt of gratitude to John P. Foreyt, Ph.D., who may not even realize just how significant a mentor he has been to me over the years. In fact, the concept for three main strategies, presented in a structured day-by-day format, was encouraged and fleshed out during a sensational dinner shared with Peter Vash, M.D., Isaac Greenberg, Ph.D., and John after a Harvard Obesity Conference session. I thank you, John, for your wit, wisdom, and continuing support.

FOREWARD

By John P. Foreyt, Ph.D.
Director, Behavioral Medicine Research Center
Baylor College of Medicine
Houston, Texas

Linda lost 163 pounds in one of our programs at Baylor College of Medicine and has managed to keep most of it off for 13 years. I once asked her the secret of her success, and she told me she works at weight management every minute of every day.

"From the time I get up," Linda says, "I plan my entire day. I eat the same breakfast–oatmeal–and drink orange juice. I eat the same lunch at Luby's cafeteria near where I work. I get the broiled fish and the broiled vegetables. I eat basically the same dinner every evening at home. I walk at least an hour a day after work."

Linda and I have an agreement. When she regains more than ten pounds, she calls me. Together, we readjust her lifestyle. She calls a couple of times a year.

Linda's maintenance of her large weight loss seems to be due to her structured lifestyle. Whenever she calls me, I know the reason–stress. Anytime she finds herself in a stressful situation, Linda's eating plan starts drifting. She begins to eat larger portions, has desserts more frequently, and starts to binge again. Stress has caused her to change her career four times. Stress has caused her to change her family twice.

In our research at Baylor College of Medicine's Behavioral Medicine Research Center, we compare people who have lost and regained their weight with those who have maintained their losses. Time and time again, we see the same patterns emerge. People who have difficulty managing stress are the ones who put the lost weight back on. People who learn to identify and handle stress are the ones who keep the weight off.

Cynthia Stamper Graff and her staff at Lindora Medical Clinics have seen the same results in their excellent weight management program. Stress is a killer. It kills one's healthy eating plan and it kills the desire to exercise. It saps people's motivation before they ever know what hit them.

How can we learn to identify, and more importantly, manage stress? This book reveals the answers. *Lean for Life Phase Two: Lifetime Solutions* is a terrific, much-needed guide for people who struggle daily with their weight and wonder why they can't seem to lose it or keep it off. Cynthia Stamper Graff, a pioneer in the field, has seen it all before, over and over. This book is a godsend for people who cannot seem to stay in control.

Lean for Life Phase Two: Lifetime Solutions takes the reader by the hand and shows step-by-step the road to long-term success. Strategies that work are explained simply and clearly. Slow changes made without deprivation are emphasized. The secrets of success are unfolded in an easy-to-follow, eight-week, day-by-day program.

In our research studies, we, like the team at Lindora, have found three essential components of long-term weight management success. These three components–problem solving, social support ("the human connection") and physical activity–are incorporated nicely into the *Lean for Life Phase Two: Lifetime Solutions* program. Each of the lifestyle modification skills presented in this program will help the reader lose weight and keep it off.

Achieving and maintaining a healthy lifestyle requires a commitment. I hope that you will make the commitment today. Read and follow this eight-week program. One day at a time. There is no better time than now. *Lean for Life Phase Two: Lifetime Solutions* is based on sound cognitive behavioral principles. It can change your life. Give it an opportunity to work for you. Eight weeks from today, you will be healthier and pleased that you did.

GETTING STARTED

If you always do what you've always done,
you'll always get what you always got.
                              -Anne Kaiser Stearns

Congratulations! The simple fact that you've chosen to read this book is a testament to your commitment to maintaining at your present weight. For some, reading this book is the next step on a journey toward better health and a better life. You may have lost weight with Lean for Life or another program and are now determined to make sure you maintain at your new, healthier lean weight. You may have lost weight many times in the past, only to regain it again and again. This time, you're ready to do it differently. You're ready to accept that even though you may know how to lose weight, you don't know how to prevent regain. No matter what inspired you to read this book, know that you have just taken a huge step toward improving your health and your life. This book offers the structure and support to help you stay the course and avoid weight regain.

When you maintain at a healthy weight, you reduce your risk factors for diabetes, heart disease, osteoarthritis, hypertension, gallbladder disease, breast and colon cancers, and depression. Unfortunately, many Americans have yet to fully appreciate the power they have over their own health and well being. According to a September, 2001 study from the Center for Disease Control, the rates of obesity and diabetes in the United States increased by more than 50 percent during the 1990s. This increase continues at an alarming rate, and researchers are noting that the increase is particularly high among children.

The increase in obesity and diabetes go hand in hand. As many as 95 percent of all diabetics have Type 2 diabetes, also known as adult onset diabetes. The primary risk factor is obesity—with 80 percent of Type 2 diabetics being obese. Diabetes is a major contributor to blindness, kidney disease, lower limb amputation, heart attacks, and strokes. In fact, the majority of people with Type 2 diabetes die of heart attacks or strokes.

The tragedy of these findings is that diabetes, like many other diseases associated with obesity, is readily preventable. The onset of many weight-related illnesses and diseases has more to do with lifestyle than with genetic predisposition.

Lean for Life Phase Two: Lifetime Solutions is designed to empower you to achieve lifestyle changes that are critical for optimum health. This is not a book you *read*. It's an eight-week program that you *live*, day by day. Over the next eight weeks, you will discover simple yet effective ways to make substantial, lasting changes in your life. This process is a powerful one. Along the way, you will actually be making physiological and neurological changes that will help your body reach a state of metabolic equilibrium so that you stay Lean For Life.

I know from personal experience just how critical it is to be proactive in maintaining one's weight. I was a teenager back in 1970 when my father, Marshall B. Stamper, M.D., was preparing to open a medical weight control office called Lindora Medical Clinic. I was one of Lindora's first patients, losing 15 pounds on the weight loss program that would later become known as Lean for Life. A 15 pound weight loss may not seem like a major accomplishment. It certainly didn't feel like it at the time, especially since I lost the weight so rapidly. The challenge, I soon realized, was *keeping* it off. For more than 30 years, I've used the principles presented in this book to maintain my weight. After my daughter was born in 1992, I applied the strategies described in these pages to quickly return to my goal weight. I have maintained within three pounds of my goal weight ever since. Now *that* is something I consider to be an accomplishment!

Maintaining at a healthy, lean weight feels terrific! For me, it's especially energizing to have my clothes fit better. And I definitely sleep better when I'm more fit. Unfortunately, the older I get, the easier it seems to be to gain weight. That's why I, like many thousands of Lindora clients, have found the program featured in this book to be so valuable. *Lean for Life Phase Two: Lifetime Solutions* can help you not only stabilize your metabolism after losing weight, it can help you can nip any weight gain in the bud. And perhaps most important, it can help you learn to eat regularly without gaining weight.

Each day of the program offers a short lesson, along with three key Success Strategies that, over the years, the experts at Lindora have come to realize are absolutely essential for weight maintenance. Over the next eight weeks, you are going to learn to "Eat Better, Move More, and Stress Less". That phrase has become a favorite mantra of many Lean for Lifers. Just this morning I received an e-mail from one of our Lindora nurse coaches (I promise you, this story is true). She wrote, "I admit I struggle with keeping myself on track with my eating plan and exercise. I hear myself talking to our clients and I generally get back on track. I currently weigh eight pounds more than my goal weight and getting to the gym has been a struggle. I'm writing to you because this morning as I left the gym,

I felt really great. I realized that when I am having difficulty, there's a phrase that always, *always* gets me focused. *Eat Better, Move More, and Stress Less*. I find myself thinking 'Yes, I can do that,' and I *can* do that. Today the challenge was getting back to the gym after skipping it for two weeks. I did it. I was able to 'move more' today. And I'll go back tomorrow."

That e-mail made my day. The Lindora associate who sent it knows the Lean for Life program so well that she can teach it to anyone. Every day she makes a positive difference in the lives of others with her knowledge and caring support. And today she'll be even stronger in her conviction that the Lean for Life strategies work–she is living proof!

Each of the Success Strategies has its own icon to help you quickly identify it every day:

EAT BETTER

Even when life doesn't allow you to eat perfectly, you can always "Eat Better", even if it means leaving one bite of that fast food hamburger behind on your plate. The awareness of what you're eating can promote better food choices. Every day you'll see this symbol and discover tips for healthier eating.

MOVE MORE

Even if you can't exercise for an hour every day (or a half hour every day, or even 15 minutes every day...) you can always "Move More"–more than you might have if you weren't so aware. Every day, you'll discover easy, fun ways to "Move More."

STRESS LESS

Stress is one of the major reasons people cite for discontinuing a weight management program. Let's face it–we live in a stressful world. But no matter how hectic and demanding your life happens to be, you can always "Stress Less", even if you can't always be perfectly relaxed. Every day, you'll learn new ways to manage the inevitable stress that life presents you.

If these three strategies sound remarkably simple, it's because they're designed to be easy to remember. If all you remember from reading this book is to Eat Better, Move More, and Stress Less, you'll be a much healthier person.

As you make your way through this exciting eight-week program, you'll also encounter several other elements designed to support you in maintaining your weight:

SUCCESS STORIES

Over the years, we've learned what works–and what doesn't–with the help of people just like you. As you make your way through this program, you'll meet people whose success strategies and stories may inspire and motivate you.

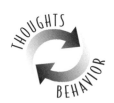

THE MENTAL FITNESS CIRCLE

Your behaviors affect your thoughts, which affect your behaviors, which affect your thoughts, etc. In other words, whatever goes on in your mind affects your body and influences your actions. With awareness and practice, you'll be able to cultivate a positive, reinforcing cycle so that you can more easily live the life you want.

YOUR DAILY ACTION PLAN

The more commited you are to maintaining a written record of what you eat and how and when you exercise, the more likely you'll be to stay aware, stay focused, and stay on track. Each day, your Daily Action Plan will help you review what you're doing–and not doing–to maintain your weight.

YOUR TURN: AN ATTITUDE OF GRATITUDE

Throughout this program, you'll have numerous opportunities to complete the following statement: "Today I live my life with an attitude of gratitude. Today I am grateful for..." Living with an "attitude of gratitude" fuels a sense of positive expectation, and believing you can do something–whether it's maintaining your weight, passing a test, or landing a job you really want–is the first step toward achieving it.

At Lindora, we pride ourselves on providing our patients with a comprehensive program that offers emotional support from professionals trained to help them lose and maintain their weight. But not everyone who is committed to achieving and maintaining a healthy weight is able to visit our clinics. That's why we created this book. We know there are many people who want a personal guide that's motivational, practical, supportive, encouraging, and always available.

So, if you're ready, this book can be your guide, day-by-day, as you enjoy the experience of living *Lean for Life*.

SUCCESS STORY: Donna Smith

Maintaining your goal weight, says Donna Smith, is like learning to ride a bike. Whenever you fall, the secret is getting right back on it and trying again.

Donna speaks from experience. Since losing 30 pounds on the Lean for Life program more than 29 years ago, the retired 68-year-old receptionist has regained five to ten pounds dozens of times. And every time, she's successfully returned to her goal weight.

"I'm not perfect, but I'm definitely determined," says Donna. "I've come to realize over the years that maintaining my weight in a range where I'm healthy and comfortable is an ongoing, lifelong process. Losing weight is one accomplishment, and maintaining it is another."

Vacations, Donna admits, are her downfall. When she set sail on a Caribbean cruise seventeen years ago, she gained 14 pounds in two weeks. Four years ago, she went on a tour to Branson, Missouri and gained eight pounds in a week. Both times, Donna immediately restarted her program and relost the weight.

Her greatest challenge, however, came three years ago when she was diagnosed with breast cancer. One of the side effects of her medications was weight gain, and during treatment she gained 40 pounds. Once doctors gave her a clean bill of health, she was determined to lose every pound she had gained.

"I felt thankful to be alive, yet I was disgusted by the way I looked and felt," she remembers. "But I knew what I had to do, and I knew I had the tools to do it."

Donna restarted her Lean for Life program and lost 42 pounds in just five months. She says her next big test will be an eleven day trip to Costa Rica later this year.

"It's a safe bet I'll put on a few pounds," she says. "And if I do, I'll deal with it as soon as I return. One thing I learned a long time ago was to never be afraid of the scale, even on days when I know I'm not going to like what I see. It's a lot easier to deal with five pounds now than it is to bury you head in the sand and realize a year from now that you've gained fifty. The secret is to stay focused–and never give up."

WEEK 1

BALANCE: The Art of Maintenance

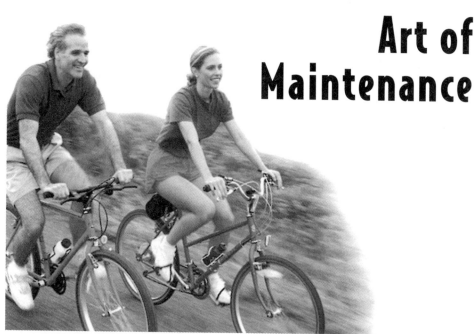

Whatever you do to maintain your weight, you want to be able to do it for the rest of your life. This week, you'll discover ways to focus your attention on the many elements of weight maintenance so you can begin balancing them in ways that work best for you.

DAY
1

"Two roads diverged in a yellow wood,
And sorry I could not travel both
And be one traveler, long I stood
And looked down one as far as I could
To where it bent in the undergrowth;
Then took the other."

– *Robert Frost*

Losing and Maintaining: And So It Goes

We all make hundreds of choices every day without being fully conscious of what we're doing. It's true that sometimes we stand at a fork in the road, knowing the path we're about to choose will have significant consequences for the rest of our lives. But for a good part of our lives, we function on automatic, unaware that the seemingly small decisions we make are shaping our destinies every day.

At Lindora, we've learned how important it is to pay attention to the details, to those "small choices". Losing weight requires, among other things, a heightened awareness of food: what, when, and how much you choose to eat. So does maintaining weight. To lose weight, you must control your food intake, move your body, and stay conscious of what you're doing so that you can make adjustments that will enhance your progress. You must also develop positive changes in the way you think – about your body, the role food plays in your life, and your general outlook. To maintain, you must do exactly the same things.

The bottom line is this: *In order to maintain your weight, you must continue all the good habits you developed during weight loss.* The only difference is that you now have a little more latitude and leeway. You can treat yourself a little more often and you can eat more, although for some people the difference between losing and maintaining their weight is just 100 to 300 calories a day.

You also have a little more flexibility to experiment with the basic components of your program to see what works for you. Maybe walking three days a week instead of five still allows you to maintain. Maybe not. The good lifestyle habits you relied on are still there, but you can employ them with more flexibility. In order to do that, you have to stay conscious about your choices.

EAT BETTER: Your Daily Action Plan

Keeping track of what you eat is a foundation of successful maintenance. If you have just lost a lot of weight, you know how important it is to be aware of what, when, why and how much you're eating. We all suffer from food delusions and selective amnesia at one time or another. ("A harmless little Caesar salad has *how* many calories?") An ongoing record helps us see what adjustments we need to make to stay within our eating guidelines.

Even if you haven't recently lost weight and simply want to stabilize at your present weight, food records are also important. One of the things that all research studies seem to agree on is that people who self-monitor both their eating habits and their physical activity are more successful at weight control than those who don't.

To help you monitor your physical habits, we've included a Daily Action Plan for each day of this program. You'll be surprised how much you can learn about yourself when you keep a Daily Action Plan. Not only will you see in black and white what you're doing–and *not* doing–but you'll also have a record of feelings and insights that will help you understand yourself on a deeper level. You'll see patterns emerge. You'll see evidence of habits you didn't even know existed, and you'll better understand how these patterns and habits either serve you–or stall you–in achieving and maintaining your goal.

To show you how to use your Daily Action Plan, we borrowed a page from Terry, a newspaper reporter who has maintained a 74-pound weight loss for more than six years. Terry writes down everything she eats, noting specifically *when* she ate and *how much* she ate. She carries a pocket fat and calorie counter with her so she can record calories and fat grams for each item. At the end of each day, she adds up the totals. Her goal is to stay below 1,500 calories per day, with no more than 50 fat grams each day. Each fat gram is nine calories, so Terry is getting 450 calories a day from fat, which is about 30%–her outer limit. (We'll explain how to calculate fat grams in more detail later this week.)

DAILY ACTION PLAN

Week ___4___   Day ___2___
Date ___6-13___   Weight ___121 lbs.___

Breakfast	Time: 7:00 A.M.	Protein Grams	Fat Grams	Carbs Grams	Calories
Protein:	2 Egg whites	7	0	½	34
Fruit:	1 c. strawberries	1	½	10.5	45
Grain:	1 Wheat toast/cream cheese	5	5	12	110
Beverage:	coffee/milk	½	0	½	4
Snack	Time: 10:00 A.M.				
PROTEIN BAR		10	5	19	150
Lunch	Time: 12:30 P.M.				
Protein:	2½ oz. tuna	15	1	0	65
Vegetable:	1 c. RAW CARROTS	1½	0	16½	70
Lettuce:	½ c. shredded	½	0	½	4
Grain:	½ oat Pita	2	1	15	66
Fruit:	1 tangerine	½	0	9	37
Miscellaneous:	No-fat Mayo	0	0	3	10
Beverage:	diet cola, 12oz	0	0	0	0
Snack	Time: 4:00 P.M.				
2 Tbsp. Peanut butter + celery		9	16	7	190
Dinner	Time:				
Protein:	6 oz. CHICKEN BREAST	52	6	0	281
Vegetable:	1 c GREEN BEANS	2	0	8	40
Lettuce:	+ SPINACH 1½ c	2	0	3	18
Grain:	½ c BROWN RICE/butter	3	2	22	115
Fruit:	1 c. fresh Pineapple	½	½	19	76
Miscellaneous:	B-B-Que Sauce	0	0	8	35
Beverage:	Iced Tea	0	0	0	0
Snack	Time: 8:15 P.M.				
½ c. NO-FAT FROZEN Yogurt		4	0	18	90
TOTAL		115½	37	171.5	1440

Today I was able to *Eat Better* by...

Cut my fat intake by:
- scrambled egg whites instead of using whole eggs.
- used non-stick spray in the pan instead of margarine

Today I was able to *Move More* by...

Increased my steps by:
- parked farther from the door.
- "paced" back and forth while talking on the phone, instead of sitting.

Today I was able to *Stress Less* by...

- Meditated before leaving home.
- Deep breathing exercises 3 times today.
- Meditated at lunchtime.

Today I feel really great about...

My new, healthy habits are feeling natural and satisfying! I feel more energetic and very optimistic!

Tomorrow I will focus on...

"WORKING SMARTER" I will prioritize my tasks and plan my day realistically.

MOVE MORE: What Successful Maintainers Say About Exercise

Physical activity is one of the habits that defines successful maintenance. Studies have shown that no matter how people lose weight, those who exercise regularly succeed in *maintaining* their weight far better than those who don't. The overwhelming majority of people who lose weight and keep it off succeed, at least in part, because they get up off their duffs and MOVE. Nearly one third of the Lindora patients who have successfully maintained their goal weight also exercise five or six times a week. One in four exercises every day.

Here are some comments from people in the Lindora program who have successfully lost weight and maintained the loss for at least two years.

- "Exercising every morning is as much a part of my day as brushing my teeth."

- "I value how my workouts make me feel as much as how they help make me look."

- "Now that exercise is such a vital, energizing part of my day, I think back on the years that I didn't exercise and wonder why? I guess I didn't know what I was missing."

STRESS LESS: Laughing Yourself Well

Did you know that emotions are built right into the human nervous system and are standard in every human population throughout the world? People who live in Berlin, Bangkok and Baltimore all laugh, cry, and get angry in exactly the same ways. Even children who are born blind develop facial expressions that are the same as sighted children.

Clearly, emotions are necessary to our survival, and expressing emotion through laughter offers multiple benefits. Recent research has shown that laughing stimulates the body by raising your heart rate, increasing brain alertness, aerating your lungs, reducing pain, and boosting your immune system. When you laugh, you increase your infection-fighting antibodies and help your body get rid of virally infected cells. Laughter can also reduce stress hormones in your body for up to 24 hours.

DAILY ACTION PLAN

Week _____   Day _____

Date _____   Weight _____

Breakfast Time:	Protein Grams	Fat Grams	Carbs Grams	Calories
Protein:				
Fruit:				
Grain:				
Beverage:				
Snack Time:				
Lunch Time:				
Protein:				
Vegetable:				
Lettuce:				
Grain:				
Fruit:				
Miscellaneous:				
Beverage:				
Snack Time:				
Dinner Time:				
Protein:				
Vegetable:				
Lettuce:				
Grain:				
Fruit:				
Miscellaneous:				
Beverage:				
Snack Time:				
TOTAL				

Today I was able to *Eat Better* by...

_____
_____
_____
_____

Today I was able to *Move More* by...

_____
_____
_____

Today I was able to *Stress Less* by...

_____
_____
_____
_____

Today I feel really great about...

_____
_____
_____

Tomorrow I will focus on...

_____
_____
_____

So the next time you have a chance to watch a funny movie, tell a joke, or recount a funny story - go for it! Laughter not only feels good, it keeps you well!

SUCCESS STORY: Carol Consolo

When Carol Consolo lost 63 pounds on the Lean for Life program ten years ago, she felt terrific. But even then, Carol knew that losing weight was only half the battle.

"Maintaining my weight loss has been a greater challenge for me than losing it," says Carol, a 52-year-old office manager. "When you're losing weight, there's a sense of momentum and progress because you're working toward a goal. What I've come to realize over the years is that staying where you want to be is every bit as important as getting there in the first place. Maintaining is a goal, too."

Carol, who now wears a size 4, says she discovered firsthand the value of daily weigh-ins.

"Several years after I lost the weight, I stopped weighing in," she remembers. "Not weighing myself wasn't an active decision as much as it was a gradual process. I got lazy. I went from weighing in every day or two to every week, then every month. Before long, I realized I hadn't stepped on a scale in six months. When I finally did, I didn't like what I saw. I'd gained ten pounds."

That experience was enough to convince Carol that daily weight checks are an essential part of her weight maintenance program.

"To me, maintenance is a mindset, an attitude," Carol explains. "I now weigh myself every morning, no matter what. It keeps me aware and focused. Anyone who has ever lost weight knows how easy it can be to slip into old patterns. There are times when I make a conscious choice to eat foods that aren't a regular part of my maintenance plan. The difference is that when I check my weight regularly, I know where I stand and whether I need to make adjustments. It's no fun to step on the scale and be surprised. I did that once, and once was enough."

Carol says her daily weight checks aren't as much about the numbers on the scale as they are about discipline, structure, and motivation.

"There's a terrific sense of well-being that comes from knowing that I'm taking care of myself and staying focused on a goal that's important to me," Carol says. "It's my way of saying, 'I like where I am and I'm here to stay'."

Your Turn.

Living With Gratitude

Today I live my life with an attitude of gratitude.

Today I am grateful for_____

_____

_____

_____

_____

_____

_____

_____

_____

_____

_____

_____

DAY 2

". . . Mental health is based on a certain degree of tension, the tension between what one has already achieved and what one still ought to accomplish, or the gap between what one is and what one should become . . . What man actually needs is not a tensionless state but rather the striving and struggling for some goal worthy of him."

– Victor Frankl

A Worthy Goal

Everything in this book is designed to help you succeed in maintaining your weight within three pounds of where it is right now. And you can do it! You can learn to maximize your physical, mental, and emotional resources to stay focused on your goal. Your thoughts and actions influence each other in subtle and complex ways: your mental attitude helps sustain successful eating and exercise habits, which in turn contribute to your happiness, and your happiness supports your resolve . . . and so the wheel turns, continuously, even over the roughest terrain.

By weighing yourself daily, you'll become acquainted with your own body fluctuations. You can account for a weight gain of up to three pounds as the inevitable ebbing and flowing of water retention, medication, or extra food consumption. But it's important to stay within this range. If there are problems, you want to catch them early. You don't want to wake up one day to discover that you've gained 20 pounds since you last stepped on a scale three months ago. Twenty pounds is much harder to tackle than two or three.

If you do find that you've gained more than three pounds, there's a sure-fire strategy to deal with it. Successful Lindora maintainers have protein for breakfast and lunch, and then a moderate dinner until they've returned to their goal weight. You don't need to feel terrified if you've gained, but you do need to act promptly and decisively.

EAT BETTER: All Foods Are Not Created Equal

It takes between three and six months to stabilize your weight. From our years of clinical observation at Lindora, that's how long it appears the weight-regulating center in your brain needs to accept your new weight as normal for you and thus reset your "set point".

Think of your set point as a weight thermostat. Just as a thermostat in your home works to maintain a constant temperature by regulating the heating and cooling system in response to outside conditions, your set point raises or lowers your appetite and metabolism–the rate at which your body burns calories–in response to how much you're eating.

So what will you eat? How are you going to make wise food choices from the multitude of choices life offers you?

At Lindora, we suggest that people in maintenance think of food in two categories: Lean Foods and Fat Foods. At first, this may sound simplistic, but it's a system that's proven successful for many Lean for Life maintainers.

Lean Foods contain less than 30% fat calories and are low or moderate in simple carbohydrates. These foods, especially those that contain less than 15% fat calories, are the foundation of maintenance eating. They include fruits, vegetables, grains, and lean meats prepared with little fat or sugar. Whether or not you can regularly eat lean foods with 20% to 30% fat calories will depend on what you discover while maintaining your Daily Action Plan. You are a unique person with a unique metabolism, and you will have to watch carefully to see which foods, especially higher carbohydrate foods, cause you to gain weight.

Fat Foods include those containing more than 30% fat calories. Foods that are high in calories from carbohydrates and low in nutritional value also fall into this category. Cookies, candy, junk food, and fast food all have to be viewed with caution. It's possible to eat more calories in a single meal of fat foods than your body needs for an entire day. This doesn't mean you should never eat fat foods, only that you'll want to keep track so you can see for yourself how your body responds. *Successful maintainers allow themselves occasional fat foods, but are very careful to set limits.*

MOVE MORE: Following Your Tracks

Your Daily Action Plan encourages you to record how active you are. We know that people who successfully maintain weight loss are *active*. They

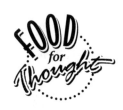

"You had better live your best and act your best and think your best today; for today is the sure preparation for tomorrow and all the other tomorrows that follow."

– Harriet Martineau

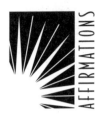

"Every day in every way, I am getting better and better."

move their bodies and see physical activity as an opportunity rather than an obligation.

In order to help you become more conscious of all the ways you can move, your Daily Action Plan has lines for recording a variety of different activities: stretching, cool down/warm up, strength training, walking, aerobic activity other than walking, and everyday activities such as gardening, climbing stairs, housework, etc. Keeping track of your activity level will help you stay active, and give you the satisfaction of watching the numbers increase as you become more and more fit over time.

Your Daily Action Plan can be a major motivator if you use it as a resource. Many people have told us there are days when the main motivation to get out and move is the simple reward of writing down their activity in their Daily Action Plan when they're finished!

STRESS LESS: When You're Smiling, the Whole World Smiles with You

Did you know that smiling makes other people think you're smarter, kinder, more confident, and better-looking? That's the finding of research conducted by Robert Zajonc, Ph.D. of Stanford University, who concluded that a simple smile can have a profound effect on the way we feel–and on how others feel about us. What's more, it can intensify our own personal feelings of well-being.

Scientists believe that when you smile, you constrict as many as 42 muscles in your face. This constriction decreases the amount of blood flowing to your brain, and thereby cools your brain. Smiling also changes the way you breathe, causing more air to flow through your nasal passages, which also cools the brain. The cooler the brain, the happier we feel. No wonder smiling feels so good!

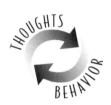

MENTAL FITNESS: The Scale is Your Friend

One of the main precepts of this book is that how you feel about something affects what you think and what you do. Your brain is interconnected with your body, which is interconnected with your emotions, forming one intricate, alive, and ever-communicating system. "Bodymind", a term coined by Candace Pert, a scientist and author of *Molecules of Emotion*, powerfully conveys the unity of this idea. As you'll discover, it's a concept with unlimited positive implications.

But there's one component of the program where we don't ask you what you think or feel it is. . . and that's your weight. That's because this is one area in which there's a much more objective measurement. Rather than recording in your Daily Action Plan what you *feel* you weigh each morning, or guess what you *think* you weigh, it's vital for you to know the number on the scale.

The scale will provide you with important data: numbers without commentary. This is not only useful, it's essential. Weigh yourself every day. People who successfully maintain their weight weigh regularly. They realize that they need to know how their daily habits affect their weight. And they're right. You can't create an eating and activity plan that's tailor-made to you if you don't know what effect you're having on your own body. The scale just gives you the numbers. It's a tool. It's one of the most effective tools you have to achieve your goal of life-long weight control.

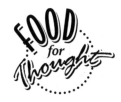

"If it were easy, everyone would do it."

— William Zinsser

Living With Gratitude

Today I live my life with an attitude of gratitude.

Today I am grateful for_____

_____

_____

_____

_____

_____

_____

_____

_____

_____

_____

_____

What is Your BMI?

Your Body Mass Index (or BMI) is now considered one of the best indicators of your risk for developing serious diseases such as stroke, heart disease, and diabetes. A recent study from Britain found that men with BMIs between 20 and 23.9 had the lowest overall risk of dying or of being diagnosed with these illnesses.

A BMI of about 22 is considered optimal for health. The National Institutes of Health considers a BMI of 25 or greater to be a risk. Individuals with a BMI of 25 to 29.9 are considered overweight, and individuals with a BMI of 30 or greater are considered obese.

BODY MASS INDEX

Height	19	20	21	22	23	24	25	26	27	28	29	30	35	40
58"	91	96	100	105	110	115	119	124	129	134	138	143	167	191
59"	94	99	104	109	114	119	124	128	133	138	143	148	173	198
60"	97	102	107	112	118	123	128	133	138	143	148	153	179	204
61"	100	106	111	116	122	127	132	137	143	148	153	158	185	211
62"	104	109	115	120	126	131	136	142	147	153	158	164	191	218
63"	107	113	118	124	130	135	141	146	152	158	163	169	197	225
64"	110	116	122	128	134	140	145	151	157	163	169	174	204	232
65"	114	120	126	132	138	144	150	156	162	168	174	180	210	240
66"	118	124	130	136	142	148	155	161	167	173	179	186	216	247
67"	121	127	134	140	146	153	159	166	172	178	185	191	223	255
68"	125	131	138	144	151	158	164	171	177	184	190	197	230	262
69"	128	135	142	149	155	162	169	176	182	189	196	203	236	270
70"	132	139	146	153	160	167	174	181	188	195	202	207	243	278
71"	136	143	150	157	165	172	179	186	193	200	208	215	250	286
72"	140	147	154	162	169	177	184	191	199	206	213	221	258	294
73"	144	151	159	166	174	182	189	197	204	212	219	227	265	302
74"	148	155	163	171	179	186	194	202	210	218	225	233	272	311
75"	152	160	168	176	184	192	200	208	216	224	232	240	279	319
76"	156	164	172	180	189	197	205	213	221	230	238	246	287	328

B O D Y   W E I G H T (In Pounds)

DAILY ACTION PLAN

Week _____ Day _____

Date _____ Weight _____

Breakfast	Time:	Protein Grams	Fat Grams	Carbs Grams	Calories
Protein:					
Fruit:					
Grain:					
Beverage:					
Snack	Time:				
Lunch	Time:				
Protein:					
Vegetable:					
Lettuce:					
Grain:					
Fruit:					
Miscellaneous:					
Beverage:					
Snack	Time:				
Dinner	Time:				
Protein:					
Vegetable:					
Lettuce:					
Grain:					
Fruit:					
Miscellaneous:					
Beverage:					
Snack	Time:				
TOTAL					

Today I was able to *Eat Better* by...

_____
_____
_____
_____
_____

Today I was able to *Move More* by...

_____
_____
_____
_____

Today I was able to *Stress Less* by...

_____
_____
_____
_____
_____

Today I feel really great about...

_____
_____
_____
_____

Tomorrow I will focus on...

_____
_____
_____
_____

DAY 3

"Health empowerment means becoming aware of–and coming to believe in–the many ways that you can exert influence over your own health and thus influence the direction of your own life. This is not just a matter of wishful thinking; it is the systematic exploration of the ways in which you can take responsibility for your situation."

– Tom Ferguson, M.D.

Maintaining Small Losses Equals Big Health Gains

Obesity and overweight are the second leading cause of preventable death in the United States today. It is estimated that 54.9% of all adults in America over the age of 20 are overweight. That's 97 million people!

People who carry too much fat substantially increase their risk of dying from hypertension, dyslipidemia, Type 2 diabetes, coronary heart disease, stroke, gallbladder disease, osteoarthritis, sleep apnea and respiratory problems, and endometrial, breast, prostate, and colon cancers. Clearly, overweight and obesity is much more than a cosmetic problem.

The good news is that *losing just 10% of your body weight* and keeping it off can significantly improve your health and lower your risk of dying from these diseases. For every 10% drop in body weight, there is a 20% reduction in the risk of heart disease. If you have recently lost weight, your health will be much better if you continue your efforts and keep it off. If, on the other hand, you have simply decided that enough is enough–you don't want to gain any more–you will also feel better and live longer than if you were to continue gaining. Either way, you're making a healthier choice.

EAT BETTER: What Should I Eat?

It's a question that needs to be answered in order for you to create a personalized maintainence program that works for you. At Lindora, we suggest that your Daily Maintenance Menu consist of:

Proteins: Three servings per day, or one serving per meal–You can choose one serving (average 100 - 200 calories each) at breakfast, lunch, and dinner. Be sure to weigh meat, seafood, and poultry after removing any skin, bone, and visible fat. Broil, boil, barbecue, microwave, roast, or "fry" using nonfat, nonstick cooking spray. Look for protein choices that are lowest in fat and calories.

Vegetables: At least two servings a day–You can choose one serving at lunch and one at dinner (at about 40 calories each). When you measure, be sure to drain water packed vegetables and thaw frozen ones. You can eat all the lettuce and leafy green vegetables you want!

Grains: Three servings per day (men may tolerate more)–You can choose three servings of bread, rice, pasta, crackers, and cereals (average 100 calories each) every day unless you find that you start regaining weight. If you start putting on the pounds, go down to two servings. Crackers can be deceptive. Choose low fat or nonfat crackers that don't exceed 30% fat.

Fruits: Three servings per day–You can choose fresh, frozen, or water packed fruit with no sugar or juice added (average 90 calories each). Make sure one of your servings is citrus.

Tomorrow, we'll talk about fat, snacks, desserts, and menu flexibility.

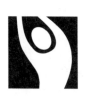

MOVE MORE: Moderate but Steady Always Wins the Race

We all know that physical activity is an essential part of weight loss. But did you know research shows that it is even more important in preventing weight regain? People who are physically active maintain their weight more successfully than those who are not active.

This doesn't mean you have to morph into an athlete to maintain your weight. More important than lots of minutes of high intensity exercise is a consistently higher level of everyday activity. You can start wherever you are right now. Walk to the store instead of drive. Walk around the block after dinner instead of watching the news. Two weeks later, you can walk twice around the block, and then three times. Many

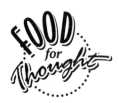

"Courage doesn't always roar. Sometimes courage is the quiet voice at the end of the day that says, 'I will try again tomorrow'."

— Anonymous

people start by slow-walking or swimming for 30 minutes three days a week, and move up to 45 minutes of more intense exercise five days a week. When you achieve this level, you'll be expending an extra 100 to 200 calories a day.

Experts now agree that all adults should aim for 30 minutes of moderate-intensity exercise at least five days a week. But the important thing is to start *somewhere*, and then to keep going. Every day, put one foot in front of the other and you'll be rewarded with greater physical fitness. Remember: the key is to *move more*.

STRESS LESS: The Basics of Relaxation

Being able to relax your body and calm your mind has profound positive effects on your physical and mental health. Here are a few simple instructions for a basic relaxation exercise:

- Make time–10 to 20 minutes, preferably twice each day–when you have privacy and are free of distractions. With our lives as busy as they are today, we need to "make time" since most of us rarely seem to have "extra time".

- Sit in a comfortable position.

- Close your eyes.

- Let go of muscle tension.

- Gently dismiss your thoughts and mental distractions by letting them float on by without becoming involved with them. Some people find it helpful to focus on a word or short phrase to repeat during this exercise, such as "one", "love", "peace", etc.

- Become aware of your breathing, and continue to breathe naturally as you repeat your focus word when you exhale.

- After 10 to 20 minutes, return to your surroundings by sitting quietly for a couple of minutes before slowly opening your eyes.

DAILY ACTION PLAN

Week _____   Day _____

Date _____   Weight _____

Breakfast Time:	Protein Grams	Fat Grams	Carbs Grams	Calories
Protein:				
Fruit:				
Grain:				
Beverage:				
Snack Time:				
Lunch Time:				
Protein:				
Vegetable:				
Lettuce:				
Grain:				
Fruit:				
Miscellaneous:				
Beverage:				
Snack Time:				
Dinner Time:				
Protein:				
Vegetable:				
Lettuce:				
Grain:				
Fruit:				
Miscellaneous:				
Beverage:				
Snack Time:				
TOTAL				

Today I was able to *Eat Better* by...

_____

_____

_____

_____

Today I was able to *Move More* by...

_____

_____

_____

_____

Today I was able to *Stress Less* by...

_____

_____

_____

_____

Today I feel really great about...

_____

_____

_____

_____

Tomorrow I will focus on...

_____

_____

_____

_____

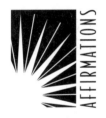

"I adapt well to new challenges."

Brain Food – The National Weight Control Registry

One of the great myths of our culture is that nobody ever succeeds at weight loss. This simply isn't true. We know from our own experience at Lindora that people can lose significant amounts of weight and keep it off. And now there is an on-going national study that also bears this out.

People who have lost at least 30 pounds and maintained that loss for at least one year can volunteer to answer a questionnaire for the National Weight Control Registry. Here are a few facts the Registry has been able to learn from their thousands of registrants:

- *Their average weight dropped from 220 to 154.*

- *The average person has lost 60 pounds and kept it off for five years.*

- *Almost all of them had tried to lose weight before and not been successful.*

- *Most said they decided to lose the weight because of some triggering event. For men, the trigger was more likely to be a health problem, and for women, it was more likely to be an emotional event.*

- *Almost all of them said that in order to lose the weight they had to change both their eating and their physical activity levels.*

- *Most said they ate less of certain types of foods, while fewer said they ate all foods but limited the quantity.*

- *Most said they watch what they eat, particularly fat, and increase their level of physical activity.*

- *Most weigh themselves regularly as a strategy of self-regulation.*

- *On average, they don't say that maintaining weight is harder than losing. About half say that maintaining is easier than losing.*

Most important of all, these people debunk another popular myth: that keeping the weight off is a miserable endeavor. On the contrary, they say they feel good. 95% say that the overall quality of their lives has improved and 92% say that their level of energy is greater than it was before.

DAY 4

"The mind is a chaos of delight out of which a world of future and more quiet pleasures will arise."
— *Charles Darwin*

The Quiet Pleasures of the Future

Chaos is a reality of life. You may look back on your previous weight loss efforts and feel frustration as you remember your own personal brand of chaos. You may have tried many times and in many ways to lose weight and keep it off, only to regain it all. Maybe you were a devotee of that magical grapefruit diet, cabbage soup diet, or your very own "all-the-bacon-and-eggs-I-want diet." Perhaps you've lost more weight over the years than you now weigh.

The truth about these previous failures is they have no bearing whatsoever on your success now. Almost everyone who is successful in maintaining a healthy weight has failed at one point in time. In fact, your previous experience can be a valuable reminder of what *doesn't* work for you.

So here you are, ready to begin. . . again. There's no reason why this shouldn't be a turning point, a moment in your life when the chaos is eclipsed by healthy new patterns that last a lifetime. It will require desire and commitment, but aren't the rewards of a healthier, happier you worth it?

 ## EAT BETTER: What Should I Eat? Part Two

We focused yesterday on guidelines for eating proteins, vegetables, grains, and fruits. Today, let's talk about fat, snacks, and desserts.

FAT: Limit your fat calories to no more than 30% of your ideal daily caloric intake. Fat has nine calories per gram, which is more than double the number of calories per gram of carbohydrates or protein. It pays to read labels carefully and consult a fat gram counter so you know how much fat

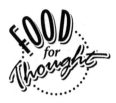

you're eating. This is especially important since some proteins, grains, and vegetables you are eating include fat calories. Also, the way some foods are prepared may add fat calories. You may be surprised at all of the "hidden fats" you discover by really paying attention to food labels and fat gram counters.

There is a lot of information available about saturated fats, monounsaturated fats, transfatty acids, etc. In an effort to keep our program simple so that it is easier to remember the basic principles, we recommend that less than 30% of your daily calories come from fat.

SNACKS: *Three protein snacks per day*–On Lindora's Lean for Life® program, people make a habit of eating protein snacks mid-morning, mid-afternoon, and after dinner. We recommend the same approach for people who want to maintain their weight. We have found from our experience with tens of thousands of patients that foods high in protein are beneficial for controlling appetite and decreasing cravings. (See the resource section for a list of high protein/low carbohydrate products.)

DESSERT (*optional*): *One daily serving*–If you decide to opt for dessert, you can substitute it for one of your daily fruit or grain servings. A four-ounce serving of fat-free ice cream or frozen yogurt containing 90 calories or less is a good choice. Learn to read food labels. What other fat-free or low fat dessert options can you think of?

A FEW ADDITIONAL TIPS TO HELP YOU ALONG THE WAY

- We base our Lean for Life weight-loss and maintenance programs on menus moderate in protein. A moderate protein diet will help you control your appetite and maintain a sense of satisfied alertness.

- On maintenance, your increased flexibility allows you to think in terms of the entire day, and not just particular meals. It's okay, for example, to eat two grains at lunch and none at dinner if you wish, as long as you stay within the guidelines for the day.

- Eat breakfast! People who start the day with a meal lose weight faster and keep it off longer than those who don't.

MOVE MORE: The Exercise Chart

As you know, movement matters. Here's a chart of common activities and the approximate number of calories you can expect to burn during each.

ACTIVITY	CALORIES EXPENDED PER HOUR	
	Men	Women
SEDENTARY ACTIVITIES		
Sitting Quietly	100	80
Standing Quietly	120	95
LIGHT ACTIVITIES		
Cleaning House	300	240
Playing Baseball	300	240
Playing Golf	300	240
MODERATE ACTIVITIES		
Walking Briskly (3.4 mph)	460	370
Gardening	460	370
Cycling (5.5 mph)	460	370
Dancing	460	370
STRENUOUS ACTIVITIES		
Jogging (9 minute mile)	730	580
Swimming	730	580
VERY STRENUOUS ACTIVITIES		
Running (7 minute mile)	920	720
Racquetball	920	720
Skiing	920	720

AFFIRMATIONS

"I find it easy to relax my body and my mind."

STRESS LESS: The Power of Prayer

In his research over the past thirty years, Herbert Benson, M.D., the father of "the relaxation response," has discovered that prayer reduces stress and promotes feelings of peace and tranquillity in those who practice it.

Larry Dossey, M.D., former chief of staff at Humana Medical Center in Dallas came to the same conclusion. In his review of more than 130 research studies, he concluded that prayer helps people overcome and prevent headaches, anxiety, high blood pressure, and heart attacks.

What may surprise you is that those who are *prayed for* also reap significant health benefits. A study at the San Francisco General Hospital

DAILY ACTION PLAN

Week _____   Day _____

Date _____   Weight _____

Breakfast Time:	Protein Grams	Fat Grams	Carbs Grams	Calories
Protein:				
Fruit:				
Grain:				
Beverage:				
Snack Time:				
Lunch Time:				
Protein:				
Vegetable:				
Lettuce:				
Grain:				
Fruit:				
Miscellaneous:				
Beverage:				
Snack Time:				
Dinner Time:				
Protein:				
Vegetable:				
Lettuce:				
Grain:				
Fruit:				
Miscellaneous:				
Beverage:				
Snack Time:				
TOTAL				

Today I was able to *Eat Better* by...

_____
_____
_____
_____

Today I was able to *Move More* by...

_____
_____
_____

Today I was able to *Stress Less* by...

_____
_____
_____
_____
_____

Today I feel really great about...

_____
_____
_____

Tomorrow I will focus on...

_____
_____
_____
_____

Coronary Care Unit found that patients who were prayed for by people they never met were less likely to have a heart attack, have congestive heart failure, need antibiotics, or experience complications.

So prayer, which has long been held to help us spiritually, is also of benefit to us physically. How wonderful!

Your Turn.

Living With Gratitude

Today I live my life with an attitude of gratitude.

Today I am grateful for_____

_____

_____

_____

_____

_____

_____

_____

_____

_____

_____

_____

DAY 5

"Every day this happens: we rotate into light. Light meets a band of earth, drapes itself simultaneously across grass and waves and trash cans, awnings and snow and mango trees, gas pumps and basketball courts and steeples and iguanas, gravestones and quarries and billboards and skin. We say of this, 'The sun has risen'."

– Leah Hager Cohen

Every Day is a New Day

Every day, as we rotate into light, we enjoy an opportunity to reclaim our reasons for wanting to live a full and healthy life. The light of our own understanding and determination illuminates our actions. Today, allow yourself a few moments to review your decision to maintain your weight. What are your reasons for claiming control over this part of your life? Do any of these possibilities ring true for you?

- I want to feel better.

- I want to avoid health problems.

- I want to look better.

- I want to feel more confident.

- I want to experience myself being in control.

- I want to enjoy my personal appearance.

Now write down your own list. The more detailed and complete it is, the more meaning it will have for you. Are you willing to make this review a regular part of your morning routine?

EAT BETTER: Determining the Number of Calories that are Right for You

It may sound ironic, but the one thing we all have in common is the fact that each of us is unique. There is no absolute rule for establishing how many calories each person needs to maintain his or her weight. Part of the adventure and the value of fine-tuning your own program is discovering what works for you now. How much food you'll be able to eat without gaining weight depends on a number of factors, including your gender, age, genetics, current weight, level of activity, and body chemistry.

There are, however, practical guidelines that will help you reach your own conclusions. As the chart on page 297 illustrates, an active man who weighs 190 pounds can probably maintain at 14 - 16 calories per pound of body weight, while an inactive women who weighs 140 pounds needs only 12 - 14 calories per pound. The chart also helps you determine how many grams of carbohydrate, protein, and fat should make up your calorie allotment depending on your gender, weight, and activity level. After you do the computation, write down the number of calories per day that will allow you to maintain your weight: _____.

The thing to remember is to plan meals that achieve a healthy balance of 45 to 50% carbohydrate, 25% protein, and 30% or less in fat. If you want to maximize your results, you can restrict your fat grams even more: sticking to a range of 35 to 45 grams per day for women and 45 to 60 grams per day for men. The calories you "save" can be used for more protein or more healthy complex carbohydrates.

When you use the Daily Action Plan and weigh yourself every day, you'll be able to see what works best for you. You will become a student of your own body and can plan your food choices accordingly.

MOVE MORE: Tuning into Your Body's Natural Signals

When Mikail Baryshnikov, the great Russian ballet dancer, was a boy, the adults around him often remarked that he was constantly in motion. His legs bounced when he sat down to dinner, his toes tapped when he talked. He ran, he moved, he waved his arms, he swung. He was alive with energy. He expressed his joy, sadness, and impatience through movement.

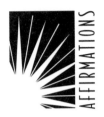

"I can rely

on my own

inner wisdom."

Even though we may not move with the grace or agility of a Baryshnikov, we still have the innate human need to move and use our bodies. It feels wonderful to bend, stretch, rotate, and to use our muscles. It's completely natural and necessary for good health.

I'm not talking about formal exercise. Routine exercise definitely has a place in weight maintenance. But right now, I'm talking about simply using our bodies every chance we get. Climb the stairs, plant a vegetable garden, carry your own groceries, walk the dog, paint the bathroom, scrub the floor, pick up shells from the beach, search for trilliums in the woods, walk to the post office, hang up your laundry outside, get up from your computer and stretch. Your body can do work, get stronger, and feel pleasure. What a gift!

STRESS LESS: Here and Now is a Good Place to Start

Through the years, I've seen thousands of Lindora patients start down the road to health by taking very small steps. One of our patients, a woman named Suzanne, began moving very slowly after many years of inactivity by walking out to her mailbox and back. A year later, she entered and finished a 5K walk sponsored by a local health organization. She says her feeling of triumph at finishing the event was equaled only by her sense of triumph at walking to her mailbox the year before.

You can start anywhere. Starting with a commitment to stabilize your weight (no matter what you weigh right now) is one of the greatest gifts you can give yourself. It doesn't matter whether you've gained and lost weight before, whether your weight has been creeping up for years, or whether you are happy with your body and simply want to stay right where you are. It doesn't matter whether you are 20 or 70 years old.

When you start taking care of yourself now, you know you'll be happier and healthier one year from now, and five years from now, than if you had done nothing. It is *never, ever* too late. A wonderful thing happens when we take *action*. We feel better, more in control, and less stressed!

DAILY ACTION PLAN

Week _____ Day _____

Date _____ Weight _____

Breakfast Time:	Protein Grams	Fat Grams	Carbs Grams	Calories
Protein:				
Fruit:				
Grain:				
Beverage:				
Snack Time:				
Lunch Time:				
Protein:				
Vegetable:				
Lettuce:				
Grain:				
Fruit:				
Miscellaneous:				
Beverage:				
Snack Time:				
Dinner Time:				
Protein:				
Vegetable:				
Lettuce:				
Grain:				
Fruit:				
Miscellaneous:				
Beverage:				
Snack Time:				
TOTAL				

Today I was able to *Eat Better* by...

_____
_____
_____
_____

Today I was able to *Move More* by...

_____
_____
_____
_____

Today I was able to *Stress Less* by...

_____
_____
_____
_____

Today I feel really great about...

_____
_____
_____
_____

Tomorrow I will focus on...

_____
_____
_____
_____

DAY
6

"We cannot do great things in this world, we can only do small things with great love. . . Be faithful in small things because it is in them that your strength lies. . . Do not think that love, in order to be genuine, has to be extraordinary. What we need is to love without getting tired."

– Mother Teresa

Without Getting Tired

In a broader context, maintenance means doing what you need to do to keep yourself in healthy balance, both internally and with your environment. When in balance, your body works well and gives you pleasure. Your mind is active and fuels your desire to learn and do more. Your spirituality allows you to discover and appreciate the beauty and meaning in your everyday life.

As it relates to weight management, maintenance means stabilizing your weight where it is right now. At first, this may sound like a very foreign concept. But there isn't as much difference between these two definitions of maintenance as you might think. In order to keep your weight steady over a long period of time–especially if this weight is new for you–it's important for you to achieve some degree of balance between discipline and indulgence, between your obligations and your desires. Staying balanced and focused is as important to maintaining your weight as it is in any other area of your life.

This program is designed to provide you with all the tools you'll need to achieve–and maintain–this new balance of body, mind, and spirit. You'll discover how to become a student of your own life, to observe honestly how you feel, how you behave, and to clarify what you really want. You'll learn how to keep track of your progress so that you can trace your body's changes back to specific actions. You'll even find yourself paying attention to aspects of your life that weight control programs usually ignore.

Most important, this book will help you pace yourself and learn to take it slowly and steadily so you don't get tired, overwhelmed, or burned out. After all, maintenance is a process, one that you'll accomplish one day at a time for the rest of your life.

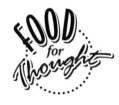

EAT BETTER: Your Calorie Bank Account

You know by now that you can't maintain your weight by consuming unlimited calories. Most of us have been there and done that at some point in our lives, only to find ourselves heavier and more frustrated than we ever imagined.

Yesterday, you calculated a formula for how many calories you need in order to maintain your weight. Once you've determined that number, you can plan to get approximately 45-50% of your allotment from carbohydrates, 25% from protein, and the rest from fat. Now you know the limits within which you want to eat.

Think of your calorie allotment as income. You have so much to spend every day. If you stay within your limit, life is sweet and the future is rosy. If, on a particular day, you want to spend less, then you have given yourself a choice. You can view the deficit as a deposit toward weight loss, or you can view it as a deposit toward savings from which you can borrow later. In other words, you can eat less one day in anticipation of eating more at your next meal or the next day.

Let's say your boss has invited you to an elegant dinner. You may want to allow yourself some flexibility for the event by eating less during that day or the following day. You could even have a "protein day" the next day. (Day 10 fully explains the benefits of a "protein day.") The point is that the average for the two days is right where you want it to be. Keeping track of calories in this way allows you some flexibility while keeping you on track.

"You can't cross a chasm in two steps."

— Rashi Fein

MOVE MORE: Put Your Heart into It

Research shows that people who include physical activity in their weight-loss programs are more likely to keep their weight off than those who only change their diet.

Moving and using your body increases the number of calories your body uses and promotes the loss of body fat. But in addition to all these benefits, when you exercise, you strengthen your heart. Whenever you climb the stairs or walk around the track, you are training your heart muscle to do more work than it has done before. A stronger heart pumps even more oxygen-rich blood to your other muscles, helping them to become stronger, too.

STRESS LESS: Creating Beauty Everywhere

Most of us are very responsive and reactive to our surroundings. Certain places make us feel good. We can sense it in our bodies when a building, a room, a corner, or a natural setting contains the kind of light and color that make us feel comfortable and relaxed. Ancient architects knew this and designed sacred spaces such as Chartres Cathedral in France and The Dome of the Rock in Jerusalem according to the tenants of sacred geometry.

You've probably had the experience of walking into someone's home and instantly feeling relaxed, comfortable, and at peace. You've undoubtedly had the opposite experience of walking into spaces that made you feel anxious, edgy, and uptight. There is an almost mystical transfer of energy and feeling.

How do you feel about your own spaces, the places where you live and work? Most likely, you can't make structural changes to raise ceilings, let in more light, or enlarge rooms. But there are elements in your private space that you can control.

Observe how you feel when you wake up in your bedroom or have coffee in your kitchen. How do you feel when you enter your workspace? Are you energized, optimistic, and delighted, or do you feel depressed, annoyed, or oppressed?

Ask yourself what changes you can make to feel better in your own surroundings. Often, all we need to do is clean up and organize. But it's also fun to see what other changes you can make to your environment for little or no money. Fresh flowers can make an amazing difference. Try framing that print, adding a spot of color, rearranging the furniture, washing the windows, displaying a favorite photograph, or making room to display a collection of something you value. The possibilities are endless.

We have been born into a beautiful world. See what you can do to keep your sense of beauty alive and well in the spaces of your life.

DAILY ACTION PLAN

Week _____ Day _____

Date _____ Weight _____

Breakfast	Time:	Protein Grams	Fat Grams	Carbs Grams	Calories
Protein:					
Fruit:					
Grain:					
Beverage:					
Snack	Time:				
Lunch	Time:				
Protein:					
Vegetable:					
Lettuce:					
Grain:					
Fruit:					
Miscellaneous:					
Beverage:					
Snack	Time:				
Dinner	Time:				
Protein:					
Vegetable:					
Lettuce:					
Grain:					
Fruit:					
Miscellaneous:					
Beverage:					
Snack	Time:				
TOTAL					

Today I was able to *Eat Better* by...

_____
_____
_____
_____

Today I was able to *Move More* by...

_____
_____
_____
_____

Today I was able to *Stress Less* by...

_____
_____
_____
_____

Today I feel really great about...

_____
_____
_____
_____

Tomorrow I will focus on...

_____
_____
_____
_____

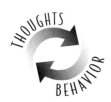

MENTAL FITNESS: Finding a Peaceful Place–A Simple Imagery Exercise

The program outlined in this book is one which supports you in taking better care of yourself in every way. Today, you'll get acquainted with a healing technique that can cause physiological changes in your body, open you up to psychological insight, and increase your emotional awareness. Along with the simple relaxation exercise outlined on Day 3, it teaches you how to use your mental skills to benefit your "bodymind." Here's how to do it.

Allow yourself to sit comfortably in a place where you will be undisturbed for ten to fifteen minutes. Close your eyes and take a few deep, easy breaths. Every time you exhale, let go of tension in one part of your body until you are completely relaxed. As you continue breathing naturally and easily, begin to focus on an image of a peaceful place that is totally safe and comfortable for you. Your peaceful place can be indoors or outdoors. It can be a place you have actually been to, or it can be a product of your imagination. Take your time to see, touch, smell, and hear everything you can in this scene. In your imagination, you can feel the air, see the colors, and run your fingers over the surfaces. Let yourself experience the deep sense of serenity and happiness that you feel by being here. Let yourself stay in your peaceful place for at least five minutes and then gradually come back to your present surroundings.

When you return, you will feel both calm and alert, as though you've just had a deep rest.

DAY
7

"The history of life on earth is an astonishing story, a tale of more than 3,500 million years. Consider what has happened since the death of Napoleon: the interpretations, the parade of historical facts, the controversies; and it will be obvious that a history more than ten million times as long can never be known, even in outline."

– Richard Fortey

Time

Compared to the great stretches of time used to describe the universe, our own life spans are infinitesimally brief. Yet it can seem to us that doing something consistently every day for the next 20 or 30 years requires more focus, discipline, and effort than we can bear. Most of us can think in terms of hours, days, weeks, perhaps even months. But beyond that, we tend to falter.

It's essential that we increase our ability to think in larger spans of time in order to maintain ourselves as lean and healthy people. We must stop thinking about eating better for the next few months, or practicing mental fitness just for the next few weeks, and cultivate ways to live that will work for us today, tomorrow, and for the rest of our lives.

True maintenance is lifetime maintenance. Short-term maintenance is a contradiction in terms. There will never be a time when you can go back to uncontrolled eating and sedentary habits without paying a price. You've done the hard work of pushing through the barriers that held you in these unhealthy patterns. Now you must think big and fuel your energy and enthusiasm for a walk into the future.

EAT BETTER: Counting Fat Grams

Most successful maintainers count fat grams so that they know how much fat is in the foods they eat.

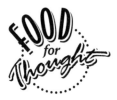

"Man, like a bridge,
was designed to carry
the load of the
moment, not the
combined weight of a
year all at once."

— William A. Ward

Every gram of fat has nine calories, more than twice the number of calories per gram of protein or carbohydrate. The average American consumes 80 to 100 grams of fat each day, which is the equivalent of about nine tablespoons of butter and 720 to 900 calories! At Lindora, we recommend one-half to one-third of this amount.

Let's say you have decided that in order to maintain your weight, you want to take in 1,500 calories a day. If you have decided to stay within the 30%-of-calories-from-fat guideline, then you would want to get no more than 450 of your calories from fat, or 50 grams of fat every day.

1,500 x .30 (30 percent) = 450 calories from fat
450 ÷ 9 calories per gram of fat = 50 grams of fat

If you've decided to get only 20% of your calories from fat, you would do the calculation this way:

1,500 x .20 = 300 calories from fat
300 ÷ 9 calories per gram of fat = 33 grams of fat

In order to manage your maintenance, you will want to become knowledgeable about how much fat is in your diet. Food labels now give you that information. In addition, you may also want to make your life easier by purchasing a fat and calorie counter to carry with you during the day.

MOVE MORE: You Get to Choose How to Move

It used to be that people had many fewer options about how (and whether) to move and use their bodies. They moved in order to work, and they worked to stay alive. Back-breaking 14-hour-a-day labor ensured that most people weren't faced with the challenge of how to get enough exercise.

Today, few of us do physical labor. We enjoy the privilege of asking ourselves what kind of exercise we prefer, and what works best for our individual lifestyles. From a historical perspective, being able to choose is a great luxury.

Aside from taking all those small, daily opportunities to use your muscles, how do you want to move? Most maintainers do some intentional walking as part of their Move More plan. Walking is cheap, easy, and available to everyone. It's also highly effective for maintaining weight. If you don't want to walk outdoors, head to the local mall.

DAILY ACTION PLAN

Week _____ Day _____

Date _____ Weight _____

Breakfast Time:	Protein Grams	Fat Grams	Carbs Grams	Calories
Protein:				
Fruit:				
Grain:				
Beverage:				
Snack Time:				
Lunch Time:				
Protein:				
Vegetable:				
Lettuce:				
Grain:				
Fruit:				
Miscellaneous:				
Beverage:				
Snack Time:				
Dinner Time:				
Protein:				
Vegetable:				
Lettuce:				
Grain:				
Fruit:				
Miscellaneous:				
Beverage:				
Snack Time:				
TOTAL				

Today I was able to *Eat Better* by...

_____

_____

_____

_____

Today I was able to *Move More* by...

_____

_____

_____

_____

Today I was able to *Stress Less* by...

_____

_____

_____

_____

_____

Today I feel really great about...

_____

_____

_____

_____

Tomorrow I will focus on...

_____

_____

_____

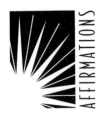

AFFIRMATIONS

"It's OK for me

to have—

and to be

— what I want."

Often, people alternate walking with other exercise for variety. They want to enjoy the activity while they are doing it and they don't want to get bored.

The options available to you these days are staggering. You can join other people and play a team sport like volleyball, softball, or basketball. You can enjoy the company of others while engaging in an individual sport like swimming, cycling, or running. You can join a gym and use the treadmill, stationary bike, stairclimbing machine, or weights. You can go for aerobics or Jazzercise classes. You can combine moving with meditation and take a class in yoga or tai chi. You can decide to build your self-confidence by taking a self-defense or martial arts class. You can decide to explore your artistic side through modern, ballet, ballroom, or jazz dancing. You can decide to take a more therapeutic approach through classes in the Alexander Technique, Feldenkreis, or Pilates.

You get to choose. Consider how much time and money you want to invest. Factor in your need for either solitude or social contact. Take a few minutes to close your eyes and ponder the possibilities. Let yourself be guided by your own needs and desires, as you find a way to take care of yourself through moving and using your body. Now make a list of at least five kinds of exercise that appeal to you. Which one will you try today?

STRESS LESS: The Glories of a Long Soak

After all that talk about playing and dancing, you may be ready for a nice, long bath. Just thinking about activity can make you want to step into a steaming bath and stay there for awhile. If your muscles are stiff and sore, add Epsom Salts to the warm water. You will feel better by the time you towel dry!

Some people have perfected bath-taking to a high art. They recognize the sensory and spiritual satisfactions of a half hour of privacy free from responsibilities and distractions lying in a warm, moist environment that smells and feels good.

Think about how you can make your bath a private oasis. Indulge yourself with candles, flowers, music, scented soaps, loofas, and big, beautiful towels. You just may discover a simple but valuable way to reduce stress, delight your senses, and reward yourself at the end of each and every day.

WEEK 2

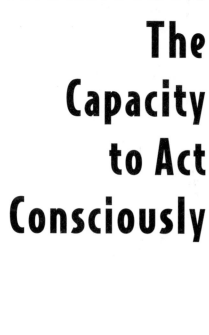

INTENTION: The Capacity to Act Consciously

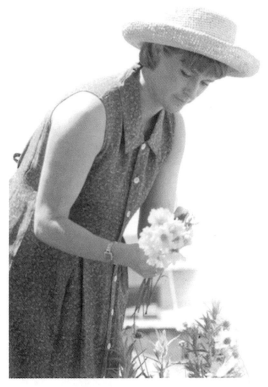

You're ready to leave unconscious, counterproductive behavior behind. This week, you'll learn how to view your behavior, your thoughts, and your feelings through the lens of greater awareness.

DAY 8

*"Tell me, what is it you plan to do
with your one wild and precious life?"*
— *Mary Oliver*

You've Already Got It!

There isn't anything in your maintenance program that is beyond your ability to accomplish. We all possess astonishing reserves of strength and understanding that we may or may not utilize in our daily lives, but which are there for us when we need them.

Maintaining your weight is an accomplishment that requires intentionality. It can't be accomplished by coasting. Our clinical experience at Lindora has convinced me of a simple truth: *When you don't pay attention, you gain. When you do pay attention, you maintain.*

Take a few moments to think about the qualities of character that are required to maintain your weight. Here are some that come to mind:

- Foresight: the ability to plan ahead and get yourself organized.

- Vision: the ability to experience yourself being successful.

- Discipline: the ability to do what you say you are going to do.

- Resilience: the ability to rebound when you get off course or experience a setback.

You may have other additions. Notice that while these qualities take strength, they are not beyond what you have already demonstrated you can do. There are no superhuman or extraordinary qualities here.

To underscore this for yourself, you might think of times when you have demonstrated these strengths. For instance, on a scale of one to five, how disciplined were you yesterday? Did you take the time to fill out your Daily Action Plan? No one is disciplined, resilient, and visionary all the time. You don't have to be. "Most of the time" will get the job done.

EAT BETTER: Moderation Over Time

Living lean offers benefits that extend far beyond looking better. You may be interested to know what The American Heart Association recommends for people who want to reduce heart disease, the number one killer in America today. The AHA now believes it's a good idea to stay within healthy dietary limits as measured over several days or a week, instead of just daily. This allows people more flexibility. You can have an occasional Italian high fat dinner or French dessert, as long as you restrict your calories for several days thereafter. They recommend no more than 30% of your calories come from fat, keeping saturated fat intake to less than 10% of total calories and daily cholesterol intake to 300 milligrams.

MOVE MORE: Overcoming Fear

Fear is distrust of something or someone outside ourselves. Although it may not feel like it, we almost always generate our own fear through our own thoughts or beliefs. *We scare ourselves unnecessarily much more often than we actually have reason to be afraid.* If you are unsure about this, observe yourself closely for awhile, and the next time you are afraid, ask yourself where the fear is coming from. Most likely, it is coming from your own ideas and thoughts.

Once you know this, you are free to gain greater mastery over yourself. You need not be enslaved to your own fleeting thoughts about what might happen. A reasonable place to start exercising your freedom is with regard to your physical activity. Ask yourself whether you are afraid of becoming active or learning a new physical skill or trying a new way to exercise.

A common fear for people who are just beginning an exercise program is the fear of being active in public. It's a shame that a fear of looking ridiculous or inadequate can rob people of the benefits of working out in a gym or walking in public. What are *you* afraid of? When you understand that you made the fear and that you can unmake it, you are free to face it, realize that it is your own creation, and take steps to overcome it.

DAILY ACTION PLAN

Week _____   Day _____

Date _____   Weight _____

Breakfast Time:	Protein Grams	Fat Grams	Carbs Grams	Calories
Protein:				
Fruit:				
Grain:				
Beverage:				
Snack Time:				
Lunch Time:				
Protein:				
Vegetable:				
Lettuce:				
Grain:				
Fruit:				
Miscellaneous:				
Beverage:				
Snack Time:				
Dinner Time:				
Protein:				
Vegetable:				
Lettuce:				
Grain:				
Fruit:				
Miscellaneous:				
Beverage:				
Snack Time:				
TOTAL				

Today I was able to *Eat Better* by...

_____

_____

_____

_____

Today I was able to *Move More* by...

_____

_____

_____

Today I was able to *Stress Less* by...

_____

_____

_____

_____

Today I feel really great about...

_____

_____

_____

_____

Tomorrow I will focus on...

_____

_____

_____

_____

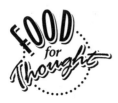

"Losing weight—and
keeping it off—has at
least as much to do
with what we put in
our minds as
what we put
in our mouths."

— Marshall B. Stamper, M.D.

STRESS LESS: Music is Good Medicine

Anyone who has ever listened to Pachelbel's Canon or a Billie Holliday torch song would have to agree that music affects mood. You're likely to feel one way when listening to a Bach prelude and quite another while dancing to the beat of Madonna.

Researchers have confirmed in the laboratory what all of us know intuitively. Music reduces tension and anxiety. Changes in heart rate, blood pressure, breathing rhythm, and hormone levels can be monitored and measured in those listening to different kinds of music.

This has great medical significance. Patients undergoing cataract or dental surgery find themselves less anxious and needing less sedation when relaxing music is played throughout the procedure. Mothers who deliver babies with music playing in the background seem to feel more relaxed. Cancer patients who listen to music report less pain.

You possess the power to use music to calm yourself and put yourself in whatever mood you desire. If you haven't already, start paying attention to how different kinds of music affect you. And then use what you've learned to choose your own special music to help you do what you need to do.

DAY
9

"Life," said Joe Butensky,
"is like a glass of tea."
If you asked him why,
"How do I know?" he would say.
"Am I a philosopher?"

– Louis Simpson

A Valuable Philosophy

Like Joe Butensky, you may not consider yourself a philosopher. But it's helpful to have an overall philosophy and understanding of how you're going to meet the important challenges in your life. Fortunately, your philosophy doesn't have to be complicated. In fact, simpler is usually better.

Let's take a look at maintenance, for example. It's helpful for people to think in terms of establishing habits that will sustain them and bring them pleasure forever, not just for a brief period of time. There is no set period of time called maintenance. You can maintain a change in your health and weight for a lifetime. That's why we recommend that you "live" this book. Read it and reread it as often as you need to. The principles you'll learn here should not lose their significance when repeated. In fact, many people report they discover something new each time they review the material.

What you're aiming for is a balance of self-control and relaxation. You want to eat enough of what you enjoy so that you're not obsessed with food and don't feel deprived. You want to enjoy the benefits of a strong, working body without wearing yourself out. And you want to establish a positive internal climate to help you meet the challenges of everyday living without feeling as though you're constantly striving rather than simply enjoying.

Having these ends in mind is important, even if you aren't there yet. You don't have to have all this figured out today. You'll figure it out little by little, one day at a time. If you pay attention, your life will teach you how to establish the right balance, and develop the strength you need to make good things happen.

So, today, as you go about your business, ask yourself these questions: What did you learn about the way you eat? What did you learn about the way you move? Be alert to what your life is teaching you.

 ## EAT BETTER: Three Squares a Day

You'll notice as you read this book that consistency is one of the foundations of successful weight maintenance. Being consistent in a moderate way is far more effective than being superhuman occasionally.

If you lost weight by following the Lean for Life® program, you know that at Lindora we recommend eating three meals a day every day at about the same time. It's also important to eat a mid-morning, mid-afternoon, and after-dinner snack to keep you from getting too hungry. You know from experience that if you skip a meal, you'll get hungry enough to eat anything in sight. In fact, you may end up consuming even more fat and more calories than if you hadn't skipped at all.

 ## MOVE MORE: Small, Achievable Goals

The secret to long-term success is to keep up your good habits forever, one day at a time. Setting small, achievable goals will help you do that. It makes sense to spend a few minutes every morning writing down or reviewing your maintenance goals for the day. Make your goals small enough to accomplish and big enough to matter, and specific enough to easily know when you've accomplished them.

If you wrote down "relax more," that might be useful in a general way. If, however, you wrote down "do two 10 minute relaxation sessions today," you would either be able to check it off at the end of the day or you wouldn't. You would be clear as to whether or not you'd achieved your goal.

Steve is a big believer is setting these kinds of goals. A successful maintainer who lost 59 pounds nearly four years ago, his typical "To Do" list includes:

- weigh in

- 30 minute walk before work

- bring tuna for lunch

- rehearse saying no to dessert before restaurant dinner tonight

- in bed by 9:30

Individually, none of these "to do's" may seem life-altering. But done consistently over a long period of time, the patterns of behavior have indeed changed Steve's life for the better.

STRESS LESS: Beyond the Self

All of the world's great spiritual programs share a common goal: to help the individual move beyond the narrow confines of the self. It is true, of course, that there are times when focusing on one's own thoughts and desires is healthy, necessary, and appropriate. Self-assessment and self-awareness are essential, for example, when you are undertaking a program of self-change such as weight loss or weight maintenance. People who live deeply contented and healthy lives, however, always say that caring for people, ideas, and things beyond themselves is both natural and necessary.

As a step in this direction, try doing something simple to care for your own neighborhood. As you take your walk today, carry a sack with you and pick up any litter you find along the way. It's a simple gesture, but one that will make a difference–not to mention make you feel good. So cut a clean swath. Make your world a cleaner, better place today as you pass through it.

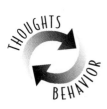

MENTAL FITNESS: A Visualization for Maintaining a Strong, Lean Body

Last week on Day 6, you were introduced to a visual imagery exercise for experiencing a peaceful place. Today, let's do a simple visualization for experiencing yourself at your lean body weight and/or ideal body shape.

Set side about 15 minutes for this session at a time when you know you will not be disturbed. Settle in a comfortable position, with your eyes closed. Take a few slow deep breaths, letting go of muscle tension each time you exhale. Continue to breathe easily and naturally as you begin to

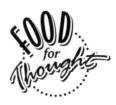

"Limited expectations yield only limited results."

— Susan Laurson Willig

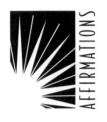

"I feel inner

peace

every day."

focus on your body at its lean, healthy weight. Let yourself paint a mental picture of your body with as many senses as you can, so that you can actually experience what it is like to live inside this wonderful body of yours. Take your time to see what your face, arms, torso, legs, and backside look like. Notice what your skin and your muscles feel like when you touch them. Experience yourself walking or running, or moving freely with strength, flexibility, and endurance. Enjoy this experience in as much detail as you can until you decide to return to your present reality.

Your Turn.

Living With Gratitude

Today I live my life with an attitude of gratitude.

Today I am grateful for_____

_____

_____

_____

_____

_____

_____

_____

_____

_____

_____

_____

DAILY ACTION PLAN

Week _____   Day _____

Date _____   Weight _____

Breakfast	Time:	Protein Grams	Fat Grams	Carbs Grams	Calories
Protein:					
Fruit:					
Grain:					
Beverage:					
Snack	Time:				
Lunch	Time:				
Protein:					
Vegetable:					
Lettuce:					
Grain:					
Fruit:					
Miscellaneous:					
Beverage:					
Snack	Time:				
Dinner	Time:				
Protein:					
Vegetable:					
Lettuce:					
Grain:					
Fruit:					
Miscellaneous:					
Beverage:					
Snack	Time:				
TOTAL					

Today I was able to *Eat Better* by...

_____

_____

_____

_____

Today I was able to *Move More* by...

_____

_____

_____

_____

Today I was able to *Stress Less* by...

_____

_____

_____

_____

Today I feel really great about...

_____

_____

_____

_____

Tomorrow I will focus on...

_____

_____

_____

_____

DAY 10

"High self-esteem provides the power to know what and who we are. It gives us the courage to live out that very personal knowledge in our daily actions, choices and ways of interacting with the world."

– Marsha Sinetar

Be Forewarned and Be Prepared

You don't have to be a Boy Scout to be prepared. But you do have to learn from your own experience. All of us have external situations and conditions that trigger temptation and old food habits. Recognizing what they are can be a real lifesaver.

Let's say you want to eat everything in sight whenever you get overly tired. If you don't make the connection between your fatigue and overeating, you'll continue inhaling candy bars and cheeseburgers on your way home from work, never cluing into a behavior pattern that's responsible for adding unwanted pounds. If you do make the connection, you'll plan ahead, perhaps packing a protein bar that you can nibble on during the your afternoon commute, taking more naps, or getting to bed a little earlier.

Let's say you become an unconscious eater at social gatherings. You leave every party you attend feeling bloated and overly stuffed. If you make the connection, you'll do a little preparation in advance. You'll eat something on your food plan before leaving home for the party. Maybe you'll spend a few moments mentally rehearsing your controlled eating behavior before being faced with all those choices. Perhaps you'll write a short statement in your diary expressing why it's important to you to maintain your weight and eat in ways that will promote your goal.

If you deal with interpersonal conflict by eating to appease your anger or deaden uncomfortable feelings, you can consciously make an effort to do something else whenever you're feeling angry, disappointed, or depressed.

Just because an old pattern is familiar doesn't mean it's etched in stone. You are a competent, resourceful person. You can change your response to almost any situation if you stay conscious and stay focused.

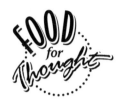

EAT BETTER: Consider a "Protein Day"

People who maintain a lean weight have an arsenal of strategies for managing their eating. Many people who have succeeded on the Lean for Life® program designate every Monday as their "Protein Day". Instead of eating regular meals, they consume six or more protein portions throughout the day, or they have protein for breakfast and lunch, followed by a small dinner of protein, vegetable, and salad. High quality protein products are high in protein, low in calories and carbohydrates, and are specially formulated to meet necessary nutritional requirements. In addition, they require little or no preparation, are relatively inexpensive, and can be taken anywhere.

A "Protein Day" or a low fat , low-calorie (1,000 calories or less) day every Monday acts like an insurance policy in that it helps correct for slips that may have occurred during the weekend.

This is the kind of food habit that can become completely routine. After several months, you won't even think about it. You'll simply have the pleasure of knowing you've developed a habit that helps keep you on track.

If the scale tells you that you are maintaining just fine, keep in mind that you always have the option of a "protein meal" when you find you've exceeded your calorie and fat allotment on any particular day.

MOVE MORE: Becoming a "Mover" and a "Shaker"

You'd probably be surprised to discover how many of the joggers you see on the street and how many of the well-defined, in-shape men and women you see at the gym were once inactive and overweight. Not everyone was born with washboard abs and firm thighs.

Many now-active people once went through periods in their lives when gym class was torture and words like "tennis" and "hiking" were anathema. The fact is that many active people are self-made. At some point, they decided to take a few tentative steps, succeeded, and took a few more. They actually started enjoying the idea of themselves as active and vital. Gradually, moving and exercising began to feel like a natural or even essential part of who they are.

With time, you'll come to see yourself as an active, fit person, able to meet a range of physical challenges. If a friend calls to say, "Let's go hiking," you'll be more likely to say "What time do we leave?" than "I think you have a wrong number." If you were asked to write down phrases that describe who you are, you'll find yourself writing, "athlete," or "exerciser," or "a person who is physically active" right at the top of the list. Exercising will not just be what you do, it'll be an integral part of who you are.

STRESS LESS: Mental Rehearsal for Balanced Eating

Sooner or later, you'll be invited to a wedding, banquet, party or other special event that'll lead you directly into a face-to-face stare down with temptation. And just the thought of being somewhere with such an abundance of terrific food will stir up anxiety and doubts about your ability make healthy food choices. You might be afraid that you'll step up to the buffet table and not stop eating until you've grazed your way through every dip, salad, roast beef, and banana cream pie in sight. You definitely want to go and you'll probably want to indulge yourself a little, but you don't want to go off the deep end.

The key to keeping your feet on the ground is to do a little preparation in advance. Dont leave home hungry. Have a protein snack before you go. But even before that, do some mental rehearsal. Here's how.

Close your eyes. Envision the scene of the party or restaurant. Take your time to see who will be there. Notice the details so the scene is real to you. What do people look like, and what do they say? Imagine the food that will be offered to you. Feast your eyes on every delicious, high fat dish you can imagine. But instead of feeling like you have to grab everything you can, let yourself enjoy the scene without feeling overwhelmed. Feel yourself to be in full control of yourself. You are comfortable, full, satisfied, relaxed. You can choose exactly what you want to eat and how much. Instead of being driven by your hunger, you can pick and choose calmly from among the offerings. Let yourself feel wonderful about what you put on your plate and how you are eating. Experience yourself leaving the affair feeling great–happy that you went and feeling wonderful afterward about your ability to give yourself what you needed–and not more.

SUCCESS STORY: Theresa Davis

THEN & NOW

Before Theresa Davis began maintaining a daily food diary, she didn't have a clue how much, when, or what she was eating.

"I never really paid attention to food–I just ate what I wanted when I wanted it," says Theresa, a 40-year-old bank executive. "My co-workers would bring lunch back to the office and I'd eat whatever they put on my desk. There were days when I was so busy that I couldn't remember at the end of the day if I'd eaten lunch, much less what or how much."

That total lack of attention to detail, Davis admits, undoubtedly contributed to her weight problem in the first place. When Theresa started her Lean for Life program, she weighed 210 pounds and wore a size 20 dress. Having made the decision to become Lean for Life, she was determined to do whatever it took to succeed. She began maintaining a Daily Action Plan her first day on the program, a habit she continues to this day.

"For me, the Daily Action Plan is one of the most valuable tools of the program," says Theresa. "As I wrote down everything I ate, I began to see patterns emerge. I lost 68 pounds, yet I ate more food than I ever had when I was fat. What changed were my choices and my level of awareness."

What hasn't changed, Theresa says, is her continued commitment to maintaining a Daily Action Plan.

"It's a tool that helps keep me accountable and conscious of how I'm eating, what I'm eating, when I'm eating, and why I'm eating," says Theresa, who today wears a size 8. "Even though my goal now is to maintain my weight rather than lose it, the information the food diary provides is still valuable. It keeps me honest."

Not too long ago, Theresa's seven-year-old son asked her whether she was going to have to keep a food diary forever.

"I told him it wasn't something I had to do, but something I want to do because it helps me look and feel good," she says. "I think that conversation was a great lesson for both of us. I explained to him that it was about results. There's great value in setting a goal and exercising discipline to achieve it, and that's what my food diary helps me do."

Your Turn   ## Living With Gratitude

Today I live my life with an attitude of gratitude.

Today I am grateful for_____

_____

_____

_____

_____

_____

_____

_____

_____

_____

_____

DAILY ACTION PLAN

Week _____   Day _____

Date _____   Weight _____

Breakfast	Time:	Protein Grams	Fat Grams	Carbs Grams	Calories
Protein:					
Fruit:					
Grain:					
Beverage:					
Snack	Time:				
Lunch	Time:				
Protein:					
Vegetable:					
Lettuce:					
Grain:					
Fruit:					
Miscellaneous:					
Beverage:					
Snack	Time:				
Dinner	Time:				
Protein:					
Vegetable:					
Lettuce:					
Grain:					
Fruit:					
Miscellaneous:					
Beverage:					
Snack	Time:				
TOTAL					

Today I was able to *Eat Better* by...

_____
_____
_____
_____
_____

Today I was able to *Move More* by...

_____
_____
_____
_____

Today I was able to *Stress Less* by...

_____
_____
_____
_____
_____

Today I feel really great about...

_____
_____
_____

Tomorrow I will focus on...

_____
_____
_____

DAY 11

"Listen to the MUSTN'TS, child,
Listen to the DON'TS
Listen to the SHOULDN'TS
The IMPOSSIBLES, the WON'TS
Listen to the NEVER HAVES
Then listen closely to me–
Anything can happen, child,
ANYTHING can be."

— *Shel Silverstein*

Developing Self-Esteem

High self-esteem is a personal strength that will help you achieve your goals in every part of your life. It will certainly help you master the skills and attitudes that will allow you to be Lean for Life.

Although some people seem to be born feeling good about themselves, most of us have to invest some effort and energy in it. Fortunately, self-esteem is something you can develop over time with practice.

So how do you do it? Here are a few suggestions, inspired by Jonathan Cheek, Ph.D. and his wife, Julie Norem, co-authors of *Conquering Shyness*:

- Practice accepting compliments graciously. There's no need to do anything other than smile and say thank you.

- Practice being authentic. Take a deep breath, and decide to let your real self shine through without running a tape in your head about what other people might be thinking.

- Practice speaking up. You may be afraid that people will disapprove of you when they know what you really think. What a relief to find that the opposite is often true.

- Practice accepting your flaws and failures. Every single person you have ever heard of who is highly esteemed or unusually gifted is imperfect. They aren't successful because they are perfect; they're successful because they kept trying until they got it right.

- Practice acknowledging what you do right. Just as we're all imperfect, we all have strengths, too. Know yourself well enough to identify and embrace what they are. Own them, take pride in them, and give yourself credit for your special qualities.

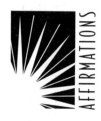

"The actions I take create the results I get. What I do matters."

EAT BETTER: Pure Water

One of the easiest and most important things you can do for yourself is to start drinking more water. Our bodies work better when we're well-hydrated. I find that drinking lots of water keeps me mentally alert and less tired. I have two full glasses of water every morning as soon as I get out of bed, even though I'm not thirsty at the time. It seems to help me get my day started right. After practicing this habit for years, I really miss my water if I'm travelling and don't drink it.

Water also helps maintain your mood at a higher level. These are tremendous benefits for such a humble habit! Although it may seem like a lot, you can easily drink 64 ounces of water a day. After all, that's only eight eight-ounce glasses. And if all that water really gets boring, you can even count herbal tea as part of your daily water total.

MOVE MORE: Moving and Mood

You undoubtedly know from your own experience that exercise elevates your mood. You can be worrying and fussing about something before you go out for a walk, and each step you take seems to melt the concerns right out of your mind. After a half hour or so, you return home wondering what you were so upset about.

A recent study from Simon Fraser University in British Columbia helps explain this common experience. Your brain makes its own mood elevating hormones, or opioids (also called endorphins) under various conditions. One of these conditions is exercise. But if you give people a blocking drug that makes it impossible for the brain to produce endorphins, they can exercise all they want and not experience the calm, pleasant feelings that usually accompany exercise. Without the blocking drug, they exercise and feel great. That's the normal cause and effect.

Consider this one of the many gifts of our innate biology. Your body wants you to take it out for a walk. As a reward you will come back feeling a whole lot better than when you left!

STRESS LESS: Your Own Calming Images

Mental images can stimulate your physical body and, therefore, affect your mental state. In just two or three minutes, it's possible to call up a mental image that interrupts your anxiety or tension and floods your body with peaceful feelings. The images that work best are the ones that are most personal to you. It can take some experimenting to discover your personal favorites. Here are some images that people we know have used to calm themselves:

- I pick up warm sand and let it run slowly through my fingers.

- I am sitting in the sun, looking into a pool of deep, clear, fresh water.

- I am bathed in a glowing, golden light that flows in and around my body.

- I am wrapped securely in a soft blanket and held like a baby.

- I am standing in an alpine meadow breathing in the clean, light air.

- I am floating gently in a beautiful, warm pool of water.

- I am looking down at my peacefully sleeping child.

Reversing the Trend

In 1991, the federal government launched Healthy People 2000, a national initiative to set goals for disease prevention. One of its primary goals was to reduce the percentage of overweight Americans by the year 2000. It hasn't worked.

In fact, the problem has increased dramatically instead of improving. Well over 60% of Americans engage in little or no exercise, and the total cost to society of obesity-related illness–and products and services that try to remedy the problem–has escalated to more than $100 billion a year.

The emphasis of public policy is now on achieving a healthy weight, rather than focusing on the lowest weight you think you should be. This

DAILY ACTION PLAN

Week _____   Day _____

Date _____   Weight _____

Breakfast	Time:	Protein Grams	Fat Grams	Carbs Grams	Calories
Protein:					
Fruit:					
Grain:					
Beverage:					
Snack	Time:				
Lunch	Time:				
Protein:					
Vegetable:					
Lettuce:					
Grain:					
Fruit:					
Miscellaneous:					
Beverage:					
Snack	Time:				
Dinner	Time:				
Protein:					
Vegetable:					
Lettuce:					
Grain:					
Fruit:					
Miscellaneous:					
Beverage:					
Snack	Time:				
TOTAL					

Today I was able to *Eat Better* by...

_____

_____

_____

_____

Today I was able to *Move More* by...

_____

_____

_____

Today I was able to *Stress Less* by...

_____

_____

_____

_____

_____

Today I feel really great about...

_____

_____

_____

_____

Tomorrow I will focus on...

_____

_____

_____

_____

means that simply maintaining one's weight within a healthy range is just as important as efforts to lose more. By following the suggestions in this book, you will continue to move toward a healthier lifestyle, developing pride and satisfaction in a healthy body that works for you.

Your Turn.

Living With Gratitude

Today I live my life with an attitude of gratitude.

Today I am grateful for_____

_____

_____

_____

_____

_____

_____

_____

_____

_____

_____

_____

DAY 12

"Finally, couldn't we just relax and lighten up? When we wake up in the morning, we can dedicate our day to learning how to do this. We can cultivate a sense of humor and practice giving ourselves a break."

– Pema Chodron

The Winning Attitude

In order to function at your best and achieve your goals, it's essential to develop a winning attitude. This is another way of saying that you will want to learn how to maintain an internal climate that helps you reach your full potential. People who excel in any arena–sports, business, politics, education, the arts–possess a winning outlook and attitude.

WINNERS ARE:

- *High energy.* Winners are physically rested and carried along by their own positive emotions.

- *Optimistic.* Winners believe they will be able to solve the problems and meet the challenges that life offers them.

- *Focused.* Winners are able to keep their attention on what they've decided is important, and possess the energy and optimism to deal with the surprises.

- *Enthusiastic.* Winners like who they are and what they're doing. They find pleasure in their lives and know how to have a good time.

- *In control.* Winners are in control of themselves and the way they respond to circumstances. They don't live lives free of challenges, but they can–and do–control how they react to tough times.

These are traits you can develop through intentional effort and practice. You already possess many of these characteristics to some degree. Once you decide to cultivate them, you'll find many ways to substitute optimism for dejection and energy for listlessness.

EAT BETTER: Eat More Fiber!

Fiber comes from the plants we eat. Insoluble fiber decreases the risk of colon cancer and other gastrointestinal problems like constipation. Soluble fiber helps lower blood cholesterol.

Fruits, vegetables, and whole grains are rich sources of fiber. Legumes (beans, peas, lentils, and peanuts) are especially good sources of fiber. Breakfast cereals can also be a good source. Look for bran cereals, shredded wheat, and low fat granolas. Read labels to be sure you aren't getting too much sugar or fat along with the high level of fiber your body needs. The recommended daily allowance for fiber is 25 grams. How much fiber do you get in a typical day? By reading labels, you can figure it out. If your fiber intake is low, which high fiber foods can you add to your diet to boost it?

MOVE MORE: 10,000 Steps

What is 10,000 Steps? It sounds mythical, and in a way it is. It's the magic number that defines for us what it means to be an active person. At Lindora, staff and patients alike set 10,000 steps every day as an activity goal.

How can you know how many steps you are taking over the course of a day? By using a pedometer. This is a small device, worn on your belt or on your shoe, that counts every step you take as you go about your day, not just when you're "exercising". At the end of the day you write down the number of steps in your Daily Action Planner. Push a button that resets your pedometer back to zero, so you can start over the next day.

A pedometer gives you an objective overall picture of how much you're moving. It not only keeps track of intentional exercise like walking around a track, but also remembers all those steps it took to go down the hall at work, to chase your two-year-old around the yard, or to run for the bus.

If 10,000 seems like an awfully big number, start with a smaller goal and work your way up. By keeping a daily record, you'll be able to celebrate every time the number increases.

You've heard that every journey starts with a single step. Think of that first step as the first one your pedometer will ever record.

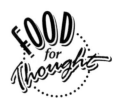

 ## STRESS LESS: A Quick Note

One of the great joys of modern technology is the invention of computer e-mail. It's now possible to stay in touch with friends and family by spending just a few minutes online every day. E-mail notes can be brief, informal, and informative. In fact, you can practically write and send a message as fast as you can think the thought.

You can also have a degree of control that's not possible over the phone. Maybe you want to send a loving note to your mother, but you don't want to get involved in a long discussion about why you haven't settled down yet. E-mail is perfect. You can say exactly what you want to say and read her reply at your convenience.

Not everyone, we realize, is plugged into the Internet. And despite the obvious advantages of electronic communication, there's still no substitute for handwritten notes. They are permanent. They can be beautiful to hold and to look at. And handwriting conveys a personal element that can never be matched by pixels on a screen.

So today, give yourself–and someone else–a loving gift by a word of encouragement, a few lines of appreciation, a sentiment that will make your recipient feel good. Whether you send it on it's way by hitting a button on your keyboard or by licking a stamp doesn't much matter. Either way, it will make a difference to the person receiving it. If you think it takes too long to write a brief note, try an experiment. Time yourself and see how long it really takes. The ten or fifteen minutes you'll spend will be well worth it. So who are you going to write to?

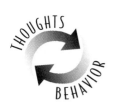 ## MENTAL FITNESS: An Affirmation for Appreciating and Even Loving Your Body

Poor body image has become a national epidemic. It's very unusual to find anyone–especially a woman–who loves her body just the way it is. Changing our attitudes requires a multi-pronged approach.

One of the simplest ways to gain more self-acceptance is through affirmations. Affirmations are simple statements you can repeat throughout the day to give yourself the positive messages that can begin to heal the damage done from years of negativity.

"Remember happiness doesn't depend upon who you are or what you have; it depends solely upon what you think."

— Dale Carnegie

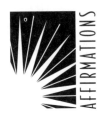

"I have confidence
that I will succeed."

Begin by listing five things you appreciate about your physical self. Write down a positive statement for each. After they are written, read them aloud to yourself slowly and sincerely, as though you mean every word. Here are some examples to get you started:

- I love my strong legs that carry me so well though my daily walk.

- I appreciate my hands and the way they let me cook, play the piano, and touch all the people I love.

- I'm so happy that my strong body is healthy.

- I am grateful for my full breasts.

If the very idea of such praise is uncomfortable to you, that's probably a real indication of how much you've been neglecting the miracle of your own body. Every single one of us possesses beauty in our bodies. Focus on what's beautiful about yours, then use it and appreciate it.

The Connectedness of All Life

We are living the fundamental miracle. The miracle is that, on earth, the basic inert elements of the universe somehow transformed themselves into living systems that can reproduce.

Most of the time, we take this miracle for granted. We forget that we are made from the same atoms that were released in that one second, 14 billion years ago, when the universe exploded into being. We are nothing less than stardust, just like the flowers at our feet, the paper we write on, or the oranges we eat.

Let yourself set aside ten minutes today to sit quietly with these thoughts. As you breathe yourself into a relaxed state, let yourself experience the miracle of your birth and your life. The same elements that are in your body are in the earth, the sky, and everything that comprises this magnificent planet we call home.

DAILY ACTION PLAN

Week _____ Day _____

Date _____ Weight _____

Breakfast	Time:	Protein Grams	Fat Grams	Carbs Grams	Calories
Protein:					
Fruit:					
Grain:					
Beverage:					
Snack	Time:				
Lunch	Time:				
Protein:					
Vegetable:					
Lettuce:					
Grain:					
Fruit:					
Miscellaneous:					
Beverage:					
Snack	Time:				
Dinner	Time:				
Protein:					
Vegetable:					
Lettuce:					
Grain:					
Fruit:					
Miscellaneous:					
Beverage:					
Snack	Time:				
TOTAL					

Today I was able to *Eat Better* by...

_____
_____
_____
_____

Today I was able to *Move More* by...

_____
_____
_____
_____

Today I was able to *Stress Less* by...

_____
_____
_____
_____

Today I feel really great about...

_____
_____
_____
_____

Tomorrow I will focus on...

_____
_____
_____
_____

DAY
13

"Always realize that there are advantages and disadvantages to every course of action. Make a full evaluation of these and turn your own disadvantages into advantages and the enemy's advantages into disadvantages."
— From *Sunzi Speaks: The Art of War*

Your Strength

It's hard to say whether there is an "enemy" to weight maintenance. Maybe it would be more accurate to say there are difficulties. And the difficulties come in many forms–some internal and some external.

People often say that they slip off their program because they get overwhelmed, distracted, and busy with other things. They eat poorly because they didn't have time to shop for healthy foods. They don't exercise because they don't have enough time. They forget to drink water because they're preoccupied with work deadlines, traffic, children, and other realities of life.

Although people don't always make the distinction, we realize the "not enough time" reason often means that work, family, and other obligations make it that much more difficult to address your own health concerns. Let's face it, weight maintenance (and other healthy behaviors) require a certain amount of time and effort.

How can you avoid falling into the "no time" trap? First, establish rituals that remind you every day of what's important to you and what you want to be doing. Get yourself organized. Each morning, write down what you intend to do to maintain your weight that day, keeping your schedule clear during exercise times, and setting aside ten minutes every day for visualizing yourself lean and healthy. Plan your food needs a week at a time, perhaps on Sunday afternoons, and find ways to accomplish your necessary tasks more efficiently. You might even consider delegating or eliminating chores you don't have the time to do.

The secret to overcoming the "no time" trap is to establish priorities and create a Plan of Action that allows time for those things that matter to you. People who maintain their weight create ways to stay focused on what's important. They don't have any more time than anyone else–they just use it differently.

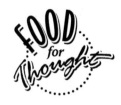

EAT BETTER: Savoring Every Bite

There's nothing quite like a vine ripened tomato, a perfect raspberry, grilled salmon, or freshly roasted coffee. From the abundance of flavors available to us every day, you would never believe that the thousands of taste buds on our tongues can detect only four tastes: sweet, salty, bitter and sour. Our brains make it possible to turn these four tastes into the thousands we discern and enjoy during our lifetimes. About 90% of the ability to distinguish flavors comes from our sense of smell.

Unfortunately, our sense of smell begins to deteriorate around the age of 60. How much loss occurs can vary greatly from person to person. But even before we age, we can blunt our appreciation for flavors by smoking, taking certain medications, eating too much, or eating too fast.

Eating is one of life's great pleasures. To get the most from this sensual delight, eat fresh foods in season, switch back and forth between foods during your meal, and slow down to savor every bite. What if this were the first honeydew melon you ever tasted? What if it were your last?

"What lies before you and what lies behind you are tiny matters compared to what lies within you."

– Ralph Waldo Emerson

MOVE MORE: The Morning Stretch

Ever notice how cats and dogs wake up in the morning with a big yawn and a stretch? The yawn delivers oxygen to the brain, and a full body stretch awakens the muscles.

Here are some suggestions for stretching yourself awake in the morning before you even get out of bed.

FULL TILT STRETCH:

1. Lie on your back, arms over your head and toes pointed.

2. Inhale deeply and reach as far as you can.

3. Hold for a count of three.

4. Flex your ankles and hold for a count of three.

5. Do three repetitions.

HAMSTRING STRETCH:

1. Lie on your back with your left knee bent and your left foot flat on the mattress.

2. Extend your right leg straight and point your toes.

3. Raise your right leg and place your hands behind your knee.

4. Gently pull forward to stretch your hamstring.

5. Hold for a count of three.

6. Keeping your legs straight, point your toes toward your head.

7. Repeat the whole process with your other leg.

8. Do three repetitions.

HIP RELEASE:

1. Lie on your back with both legs straight and your arms stretched out to the side at shoulder level.

2. Raise your right leg slightly and roll onto your left hip with the toes on your right foot pointing toward your left hand. Keep your shoulders on the mattress.

3. Return to your starting position.

4. Repeat the process with your left leg.

Tomorrow, you'll learn two more terrific morning stretches.

 ## STRESS LESS: But Someone's Got to Do It!

Nothing is quite so loving as taking on a task that you know someone else doesn't want to do. Just think of a chore you dread and imagine a friend volunteering to do it for you. Do you break into a sweat when you have to call the travel agent and book airline flights? What if your spouse did it for you? Does the thought of grocery shopping make you want to crawl into bed and pull the covers over your head? What if you didn't have to do it this week?

When you imagine the relief you'd feel if someone took over an undesirable chore for you, you can identify with the gratitude that someone else will feel today when you run that errand, or make that call, or do that household chore so they won't have to. Many of our most compelling Lean for Life "Success Stories" are those of people who tell us they "find excuses" to move more. So take the opportunity to move more and help someone else at the same time. Walk across the room to answer the phone. Take out the trash. Run that errand to the post office–on foot. Not only will it thrill the person who usually handles that chore, but it'll make you feel good and add steps to your pedometer.

SUCCESS STORY: Austin Kovac

THEN&NOW

At 15, Austin Kovac has learned more about discipline and commitment than many people twice or three times his age will ever know.

When officials of a community football league told him he was ineligible to play because he was 33 pounds over the league weight limit, Austin, who stood 5'8" and weighed 193 pounds, made a decision.

"I was tired of always being the fat kid," he remembers. "I was tired of having other kids make fun of me and tired of feeling my thighs rub together when I walked. I decided I was going to do whatever it took to lose the weight and that I was going to play football."

Within eight weeks, Austin had lost 43 pounds on the Lean for Life program. While he wasn't permitted to play in league games until he met the weight limit, his coaches did allow him to train with the team while he was losing weight. By the third week of the season, Austin had achieved his weight goal and was on the team's starting line-up as left guard.

"Losing weight is the best thing I've ever done for myself," Austin says. "It really taught me to set a goal and go for it."

DAILY ACTION PLAN

Week _____   Day _____

Date _____   Weight _____

Breakfast Time:	Protein Grams	Fat Grams	Carbs Grams	Calories
Protein:				
Fruit:				
Grain:				
Beverage:				
Snack Time:				
Lunch Time:				
Protein:				
Vegetable:				
Lettuce:				
Grain:				
Fruit:				
Miscellaneous:				
Beverage:				
Snack Time:				
Dinner Time:				
Protein:				
Vegetable:				
Lettuce:				
Grain:				
Fruit:				
Miscellaneous:				
Beverage:				
Snack Time:				
TOTAL				

Today I was able to *Eat Better* by...

_____

_____

_____

_____

Today I was able to *Move More* by...

_____

_____

_____

Today I was able to *Stress Less* by...

_____

_____

_____

_____

Today I feel really great about...

_____

_____

_____

Tomorrow I will focus on...

_____

_____

_____

Austin says the way he thinks about food has changed dramatically.

"When I was fat, I was always thinking about food and when and what I was going to eat next," Austin remembers. "I always felt sort of tired. Now, I eat when I'm hungry."

The way people treat him today, Austin says, is also very different.

"When you're fat, people definitely look at you in a different light," he says. "It may not be right, but it's a fact. Other kids would never come up and talk to me when I was overweight. They would make fun of me. That doesn't happen now. I've noticed that my attitude has changed a lot, too. I'm a lot more cheerful and self-confident."

His parents, he says, were his cheerleaders, encouraging him to stay focused on his goal. Even his grandmother got into the spirit. Instead of sending him a box of cookies as she often had, she sent a container of carrots as a show of support.

Austin says the success he's enjoyed on his weight loss program has carried over into other areas of his life.

"I'm getting the best grades I've ever had," he says. "I'm taking guitar and piano lessons, playing baseball, and doing all sorts of other things I never would have tried before. I used to be pretty lazy. I watched a lot of TV and played video games. I have a lot more energy. I stay up later, get up earlier, and get a lot more done. I hardly ever lie around the house anymore. I'm too busy having fun."

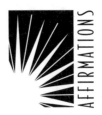

AFFIRMATIONS

"If it's
to be, it's up
to me."

DAY
14

"Watch out for the barriers to change that lurk in all our minds–nostalgia for an imagined past, lack of awareness, workaholism, arrogance, the need for control or power, perfectionism, lack of confidence, the need to be right, a closed mind, stress, waiting for someone else to change, fear of loss, grief. On your journey into the future, these are the barriers that will trip you up and slow you down."

– Jennifer James

The Art of Seeing What You are Doing Right

That's quite a list of barriers that Jennifer James mentions. They describe an attitude that is tight, narrow, and closed. The opposite is an attitude that is relaxed, open, and curious. A very important element in this open stance is a readiness to see yourself fully–not to limit your perception of yourself because of preconceived ideas, but to see yourself as the strong and valuable person you really are.

If this appreciative view of yourself is unfamiliar, you might start retraining yourself by beginning to notice the little things you are doing right. You can start right now. What have you done right so far today? If it's hard for you to think of even one thing, then go back to basics. Did you get out of bed on time? Did you eat a good breakfast? Did you remember your keys?

Soon enough, you'll get bored with the basics and begin looking for behaviors that are more significant. Instead of automatically lapsing into your litany of morning complaints, did you affirm that you were going to have a good day at work? After you weighed yourself, did you feel good about staying within your limit? Did you remember to say an encouraging word to each of your children as they headed off to school? Did you remember to write down your pedometer steps on your Daily Action Plan?

Start giving yourself credit for all the things you do right, for all the ways you are a good and loving person, for efforts you make–whether they turn out this time or not. Do as good a job loving yourself as you do loving others.

EAT BETTER: Vitamins

Vitamin and mineral supplements are an essential part of a healthy weight maintenance program. At Lindora, we've developed our own supplement that may be ordered by mail or phone from the resource section at the back of this book. If you prefer to purchase vitamins at a grocery or drug store, you may compare the labels with this ingredient list to make sure the daily vitamin dosage you take contains these important vitamins and minerals:

VITAMINS & MINERALS	SIZE	%USDA
Vitamin A (Beta Carotene)	5000 IU	100
Vitamin D (Ergocalciferol)	400 IU	100
Vitamin E (d-Alpha Tocopheryl Acetate)	200 IU	667
Vitamin C (Ascorbic Acid)	600 mg	1000
Folic Acid	400 mcg	100
Vitamin B-1 (Thiamine)	100 mg	6667
Vitamin B-2 (Riboflaven)	100 mg	5882
Niacinamide	100 mg	500
Vitamin B-6 (Pyridoxine)	100 mg	5000
Vitamin B-12 (Cyanocobalamin)	500 mcg	8333
Biotin	100 mcg	33
Pantothenic Acid (d-Calcium Pantothenate)	100 mg	1000
Calcium (Carbonate Di-Calcium Phosphate)	400 mg	40
Phosphorous (Di-Calcium Phosphate)	100 mg	10
Iodine (Kelp)	100 mcg	67
Iron (Gluconate)	15 mg	83
Magnesium (Oxide)	200 mg	50
Copper (Gluconate)	2 mg	100
Zinc (Gluconate)	40 mg	267
Potassium (Gluconate)	99 mg	**
Manganese (Gluconate)	5 mg	**
Chromium	10 mcg	**
Rutin	50 mcg	***
Lemon Bioflavinoids Complex	200 mg	***

VITAMINS & MINERALS continued	**SIZE**	**%USDA**
Inositol	400 mg	***
Choline (Bitartrate)	700 mg	**
Para Amino Benzoic Acid	100 mg	***
Selenium (L-Selenomethione)	100 mg	**

    *   Percentage of US Recommended Daily Allowance.

   * *   Percentage of US Recommended Daily Allowance Not Established.

* * *   Need in human nutrition not established.

MOVE MORE: Be Good to Yourself

At Lindora, it's our philosophy that people should find ways to say "yes" to themselves as often as they can, as long as the "yes" is healthy. Many people find it motivating to reward themselves for small accomplishments that keep them on the right track.

Let's say that you set a goal of walking 2,000 more steps per day by the end of the week than you usually do. You might want to reward yourself for reaching your goal. A new pair of athletic socks? A new tape for your Walkman? Concert or theater tickets? A massage? Accomplish a goal and create a reward that works for you.

STRESS LESS: Giving Gifts

Just as it's fun to reward yourself, it can also be a kick to give small presents to other people. Every so often, you can surprise a co-worker or a family member with something you've chosen for them "just because".

Possibilities are everywhere. A flower from your garden, a pretty pebble from the beach, a paperback book, an exotic herb from the garden shop, a new soap from the scent shop, a gift certificate to your favorite coffee shop, a new brand of tea. Your explanation can be simple: "I saw this and I thought of you." What a loving way to treat your friends–and yourself.

DAILY ACTION PLAN

Week _____ Day _____

Date _____ Weight _____

Breakfast	Time:	Protein Grams	Fat Grams	Carbs Grams	Calories
Protein:					
Fruit:					
Grain:					
Beverage:					
Snack	Time:				
Lunch	Time:				
Protein:					
Vegetable:					
Lettuce:					
Grain:					
Fruit:					
Miscellaneous:					
Beverage:					
Snack	Time:				
Dinner	Time:				
Protein:					
Vegetable:					
Lettuce:					
Grain:					
Fruit:					
Miscellaneous:					
Beverage:					
Snack	Time:				
TOTAL					

Today I was able to *Eat Better* by...

_____
_____
_____
_____

Today I was able to *Move More* by...

_____
_____
_____
_____

Today I was able to *Stress Less* by...

_____
_____
_____
_____
_____

Today I feel really great about...

_____
_____
_____

Tomorrow I will focus on...

_____
_____
_____
_____

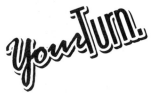

Over the Last Four Days . . .

- How many steps have you averaged? _____

- How many days have you completed your Daily Action Plan? _____

- How many days did you weigh yourself? _____

- Remember: The program works when you work the program.

WEEK 3

FUEL: The Strategy of Balanced Eating

It is possible to develop a healthy love affair with food, even if you haven't had one up to now. There is so much to learn about how to eat for maintenance. This week, you'll learn to focus on your food choices, your food feelings, and your food needs.

DAY 15

"We eat to satisfy emotional as well as physical needs, and unless both are acknowledged and dealt with, we are setting ourselves up to feel deprived and go hunting for more food."
– Geneen Roth

Creating Your Own Plan

The food guidelines outlined earlier in this book are the result of years of clinical experience combined with the best information available from current research. We know, for example, that to maintain your weight, you need to keep your calories within certain limits, exercise regularly, and weigh yourself often.

But within that structure, you have enormous freedom to tailor a food and activity plan that works for you right now. What works for you this year may not work as well next year, at which time you can choose to create a different plan. Over the years, you may find that some parts of your plan remain the same, while other elements of it may change dramatically.

Some people make breakfast the biggest meal of the day, while others distribute their calories throughout the day. There are those who enjoy having the same snacks day in and day out, and others who need variety in order to stay on course. Some of us need and want more complex carbohydrates than others. Some people vary their calorie intake depending on how much exercise they have done on a particular day. Some of us can get away with splurging on high fat treats more often than others.

People who successfully maintain their weight over the years tailor the basic food guidelines to meet their own unique physical and emotional needs. They become familiar with their own patterns of physical hunger. They know when they need to be very disciplined and when they can relax a little.

You, too, can tune into your body and commit yourself to an eating program that will sustain you for the rest of your life. The tools featured in this book will help you do it.

EAT BETTER: Monthly Cravings

Women who find themselves feeling hungrier during certain days of their menstrual cycle are not imagining things. A review of research indicates that a substantial proportion of women indeed experience real, biological changes in appetite during their cycles.

One researcher, Susan I. Barr, R.D.N., Ph.D., found that food consumption was typically greater during the latter half of a woman's monthly cycle, two to three weeks after her period. The average woman consumes an additional 300 calories a day during this phase.

If you're a woman who has noticed this pattern in your monthly cycle, try to eat as normally as possible. If you decide to allow yourself a few extra calories, pay attention to where they're coming from. Since you're weighing yourself every day, you'll know if it makes sense to balance these extra calories by exercising more for a couple of days.

MOVE MORE: Inspiration

Most of us are inspired more by the people we know than by the ideas we're exposed to. Information is important and necessary, but that fit, middle-aged woman in the office next door may do more to inspire you to get out and swim than all the facts about exercise compiled by the National Institutes of Health.

You must know someone who is already living Lean for Life. Within your circle of family, friends, business associates, neighbors, and other acquaintances, there's certainly a man or woman who's consistent in exercise, careful about eating, and wise in taking care of himself or herself. You might consider asking that person to talk with you about their own journey. How and when did she start becoming physically active? What is his daily schedule like? How does she eat? Most people who are conscious about their health are more than willing to share their success strategies.

If you look for it, inspiration is everywhere. You can learn just as much from your less obviously fit friends. The most inspiring stories often involve people who have overcome tremendous odds that most of us

DAILY ACTION PLAN

Week _____   Day _____

Date _____   Weight _____

Breakfast	Time:	Protein Grams	Fat Grams	Carbs Grams	Calories
Protein:					
Fruit:					
Grain:					
Beverage:					
Snack	Time:				
Lunch	Time:				
Protein:					
Vegetable:					
Lettuce:					
Grain:					
Fruit:					
Miscellaneous:					
Beverage:					
Snack	Time:				
Dinner	Time:				
Protein:					
Vegetable:					
Lettuce:					
Grain:					
Fruit:					
Miscellaneous:					
Beverage:					
Snack	Time:				
TOTAL					

Today I was able to *Eat Better* by...

_____

_____

_____

_____

Today I was able to *Move More* by...

_____

_____

_____

_____

Today I was able to *Stress Less* by...

_____

_____

_____

_____

Today I feel really great about...

_____

_____

_____

_____

Tomorrow I will focus on...

_____

_____

_____

_____

never have to face. Someone who's learned to walk again after a serious accident can inspire you in ways that a successful marathon runner can't, and vice versa. So let yourself be open to the lessons that others can share with you, and don't be surprised one day if someone sees you as an inspiration and wants to know how *you* became a success.

STRESS LESS: The Power of the Compliment

As you go through your day today, be on the lookout for someone you can compliment. Surround yourself with an aura of appreciation, and notice the small things that people do to add to the beauty, joy, and civility of life. And then let them know you appreciate it.

SUCCESS STORY: Sonya LaRusso

There was a time when Sonya LaRusso thought of food as the enemy–and the enemy was winning.

"I used to be afraid of food because I didn't know anything about nutrition," says Sonya, 47. "Ten years ago, I was taking diet pills and I weighed 97 pounds. But once I stopped the pills, my appetite spun out of control. I regained all my weight plus an extra fifty pounds. I was eating chocolate and greasy foods every day. I knew I needed to learn how to eat healthy if I were ever going to gain control over my weight."

Sonya, who lost 101 pounds and went from a size 26 to a size 9 in just six months, says she values the education and perspective she gained on the Lean for Life program as much as the weight loss success she achieved.

"Once I began learning how and what to eat, my body–and my life–really began to change," she explains. "My entire relationship with food is different today. The way I eat, how much I eat, when I eat has all changed."

Sonya says the way she shops for food has changed, too.

"It used to be that if something looked good, into the cart it went," she remembers. "I never read a food label in my life. But now, I pay attention to what I'm buying. I compare the nutritional values of different brands, and I make a real effort to avoid eating too many carbohydrates. The more carbs I eat, the hungrier I tend to get."

What makes Sonya's success story all the more remarkable is that she continued cooking high-carb, high fat Italian dishes for her husband while following her weight loss program.

"I would make shish kabob or pork and potatoes for him and broiled chicken for me," recalls Sonya. "But I never felt deprived because I knew the way I was eating was making a real difference in the way I looked and felt."

Exercise was also part of Sonya's grand plan. Today, she still makes a concerted effort to stay active by walking an hour every morning and doing an hour on the treadmill every night.

"It's a commitment I'm willing to make because I see results," she says. "I've maintained within two pounds of my goal weight for nearly a year now. And that's a good thing because I gave all my fat clothes away. There's no way I'm ever going to need them again."

Your Turn. Living With Gratitude

Today I live my life with an attitude of gratitude.

Today I am grateful for_____

_____

_____

_____

_____

_____

_____

_____

_____

_____

_____

DAY 16

"The first step toward becoming conscious is learning to become aware of the constantly changing landscape of thoughts, feelings, and perceptions that constipate the mind and mask awareness of the inner physician. Lost in the inner dialogue, we are only partly awake, sleepwalking our way through life."

– Joan Borysenko

Waking Up

Many of us have spent much of our lives eating unconsciously. In fact, overeating helps us sleepwalk through our lives. We learn that if we eat enough, fast enough, we sometimes can't even remember what we were so upset about in the first place. The unkind word loses its sting, and our own imperfections don't seem so overwhelming. It's easy to medicate ourselves–and salve our feelings–with food.

Making a commitment to maintain weight loss is really about making a commitment to wake up, to become and remain conscious. We no longer allow ourselves the option of eating too much, too fast. We stay awake and aware of our own discomfort and our own pain. We live through it and discover that our feelings don't kill us.

Planning what to eat and keeping track of your food is wonderful practice for being conscious in other areas of your life. You learn how to meet your own needs, how to eat for pleasure, how to find satisfaction in moderation, and how to become aware of what you are doing–and *why* you are doing it. You eat–and live–more wisely.

 ## EAT BETTER: The Special Nutritional Concerns of Men

For every 100 women who die between the ages of 45 and 64, 170 men die. Men are more likely to die from heart disease, cancer, stroke, pneumonia, and AIDS. Men are more likely to be overweight than women. A recent study found that 59% of American men are overweight compared to 49% of women. While genetic predisposition certainly plays a role in who gets which disease, how we choose to take care our ourselves clearly plays a major role.

One of the major health risks for men today is prostate cancer. Approximately 300,000 men will be diagnosed with it this year and 41,000 will die. Many studies have established a link between eating habits and prostate cancer. Here are some dietary changes men can make to reduce their risk:

- Reduce the amount of saturated fat (found in animal foods), and replace it with the amount of omega-3 fatty acids (found in fish).

- Eat soy products, such as soy milk, soy flour, and tofu.

- Eat fruits and vegetables.

- Eat beans and legumes.

- Eat tomatoes, especially in cooked form such as tomato sauce.

- Be sure you are getting 100% of your daily requirement of vitamin D.

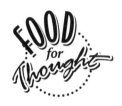

"Continuous effort—not strength or intelligence—is the key to unlocking our potential."

— Liane Cordes

MOVE MORE: More Morning Stretches

Last week, we described three stretches you can do before you even get out of bed. Today, let's look at two new stretches: one you can do while you're still in bed, and another you can do standing up.

LOWER BACK RELEASE

1. Lie on your back.

2. Bend your right leg and raise it toward your chest.

3. Grasp with both hands behind your knee.

4. Gently pull toward you.

5. Do three repetitions.

6. Repeat with the other leg.

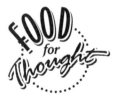

"Habit is habit, and
not to be flung out
of the window, but
coaxed downstairs a
step at a time."

— Mark Twain

THE APPLE STRETCH

1. Get out of bed and stand up.

2. Reach skyward with both arms and pretend you're picking apples from a branch just out of reach. You can stand on tiptoes if you want to stretch even more.

3. Pick first with the right hand, and then with the left.

4. Pick twenty apples in a row.

5. Lower both arms and shake.

6. Bend from the waist, allowing your arms to dangle toward your toes. Shake your arms.

7. Do three repetitions.

STRESS LESS: A Healthy Sexuality

Sexual interaction with a loving partner is a rich source of pleasure and one of the best things you can do for your bodymind. But people who have had a heart attack often harbor lingering worries that sexual intercourse will increase their risk of having another attack.

A recent study helps put those worries to rest. The absolute risk of having another heart attack after sexual activity is so slight as to be practically nonexistent. And people who engage in regular physical activity two or three times a week reduce even that minuscule risk. Consider this yet another terrific reason to become physically active!

DAILY ACTION PLAN

Week _____   Day _____

Date _____   Weight _____

Breakfast Time:	Protein Grams	Fat Grams	Carbs Grams	Calories
Protein:				
Fruit:				
Grain:				
Beverage:				
Snack Time:				
Lunch Time:				
Protein:				
Vegetable:				
Lettuce:				
Grain:				
Fruit:				
Miscellaneous:				
Beverage:				
Snack Time:				
Dinner Time:				
Protein:				
Vegetable:				
Lettuce:				
Grain:				
Fruit:				
Miscellaneous:				
Beverage:				
Snack Time:				
TOTAL				

Today I was able to *Eat Better* by...

_____
_____
_____
_____

Today I was able to *Move More* by...

_____
_____
_____
_____

Today I was able to *Stress Less* by...

_____
_____
_____
_____

Today I feel really great about...

_____
_____
_____

Tomorrow I will focus on...

_____
_____
_____

DAY 17

"When boredom arises, feel it in the body. Stay with it. Let yourself be really bored. Name it softly as long as it lasts. See what the demon is. Note it, feel its texture, its energy, the pains and tensions in it, the resistances to it. See what story it tells and what opens up as you listen. When we finally stop running away or resisting it, then wherever we are can actually become interesting!"

– Jack Kornfield

Boredom

Part of being mentally strong is developing a tolerance for boredom. It's useful in all areas of life to be able to accept those "nothing special" times when not much is happening. It's especially useful in the area of eating.

We are all trying to find a balance between pleasure–even excitement–in eating and not needing any special perks from our food at all. None of us would want to live in a world where everything we ate was dull and tasteless. On the other hand, we don't want to depend too much on the perfect meal, snack, or dessert to cheer us up. It's too easy to get caught in an downward spiral where linguine and tomato sauce does the job for awhile, but then we need to add parmesan. Soon we're adding pesto. Before long, we're mixing in a little Italian sausage.

The appropriate life-long task is how to eat so we sometimes eat for the thrill but usually eat for the satisfaction of healthy sustenance. Try getting your excitement needs met in other ways–such as living in a strong, lean body!

EAT BETTER: An Example of a High Fiber Menu

Here are some simple suggestions for increasing the amount of fiber in your diet.

- Start the day with a high fiber, whole grain cereal with fresh fruit.

- Add lentils, beans, and rice to your normal fare, or eat them in place of meat-based dishes.

- Eat fresh, unprocessed fruit. Bananas, pears, apples, and dried fruits are high in fiber.

- Eat fresh vegetables. Sweet potatoes, carrots, asparagus, spinach, broccoli, and peas are high in fiber.

- When you eat bread, make it whole grain.

- Add garbanzo beans to your salads.

- Eat air-popped popcorn as a snack.

- Eat carrots as a snack.

- Eat an orange instead of drinking a glass of orange juice.

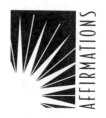

AFFIRMATIONS

"I am enjoying doing the things that are helping me become lean and healthy."

MOVE MORE: Bathroom Bonus

The notion of doing bathroom exercises may sound strange, but remember your goal: to keep moving and have fun! Try these exercises every morning for a week. You'll like how they make you feel!

TOOTHBRUSH TUSH PUSH

1. Turn on some dancing music.

2. Put toothpaste on your brush.

3. Stand tall, feet apart and toes turn slightly out.

4. As you brush your teeth, bend and straighten your knees in time to the music.

The American Dental Association recommends brushing for one to two minutes at least twice a day. That's an extra four minutes of knee bends every day!

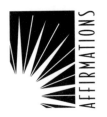

AFFIRMATIONS

"I eat to fuel
my body."

TOWEL TONER

1. Keep the music on.

2. Stand with your feet apart.

3. Grab your towel with both hands and hold it taut behind your head.

4. Bend at the waist from side to side. Twelve times to the left. Twelve times to the right.

Get into the beat and make it fun.

UPSIDE DOWN TOE TOUCHES

1. With the music still on, stand with your feet apart.

2. Bend forward from the waist and towel dry your hair upside down.

3. Use your free hand to reach for your toes.

4. Switch and reach for your toes with your other hand.

5. Do alternative intervals of eight.

STRESS LESS: Living With Gratitude

Have you ever noticed that it's often the people who have faced the greatest struggles in life who are the most grateful for what they have? Perhaps that's because they know what it means to do without.

We all have so much to be thankful for. Living with a sense of gratitude is life transforming. Here's an easy way to get a fuller picture of how lucky you are in spite of your difficulties. Review your list of current complaints. Then construct a sentence that acknowledges each difficulty, but goes on to express gratitude for the bigger picture. Some examples:

- I wish my back didn't ache, but I'm grateful I can walk. Some people can't.

- I wish I made more money, but I'm grateful that we have a roof over our heads and food on our table. Some people don't have either.

- I'm tired of the demands of my family, but I'm grateful that I'm not alone. Some people are very lonely.

DAILY ACTION PLAN

Week _____   Day _____

Date _____   Weight _____

Breakfast	Time:	Protein Grams	Fat Grams	Carbs Grams	Calories
Protein:					
Fruit:					
Grain:					
Beverage:					
Snack	Time:				
Lunch	Time:				
Protein:					
Vegetable:					
Lettuce:					
Grain:					
Fruit:					
Miscellaneous:					
Beverage:					
Snack	Time:				
Dinner	Time:				
Protein:					
Vegetable:					
Lettuce:					
Grain:					
Fruit:					
Miscellaneous:					
Beverage:					
Snack	Time:				
TOTAL					

Today I was able to *Eat Better* by...

_____
_____
_____
_____

Today I was able to *Move More* by...

_____
_____
_____
_____

Today I was able to *Stress Less* by...

_____
_____
_____
_____
_____

Today I feel really great about...

_____
_____
_____

Tomorrow I will focus on...

_____
_____
_____

- I'm tired of having to work so hard at maintenance, but I'm grateful that I have this opportunity to take good care of myself. Some people suffer daily with severe health problems they can't control.

Whether or not you feel fortunate or unfortunate is largely a matter of attitude. But you can be sure that you'll be happier and live a more satisfying life when you practice daily gratitude for what you have.

Chewing the Fat

The conclusion is inescapable. There are overwhelming health benefits to eating more omega-3 fatty acids, a type of fat with powerful health-protecting benefits. Omega-3 strengthens your defenses against heart disease, stroke, rheumatoid arthritis, high blood pressure, and some kinds of cancer.

Omega-3 is found in fish, both fresh and canned. Fish especially high in omega-3's include anchovies, halibut, herring, mackerel, salmon (Atlantic, Chinook, Coho, King, Pink, Sockeye), Sardines, Shark, Trout (Rainbow, Lake) and tuna (Albacore, Bluefin).

Plant sources of omega-3 oils are canola oil, soybean oil, spinach, mustard greens, tofu, wheat germ, walnuts, and flaxseed. Stock your kitchen with olive oil and canola oil instead of other kinds of oils.

Following these suggestions is an easy way to benefit your overall health in every possible way.

DAY 18

"Some obese people are unable to tell the difference between being scared, angry, and hungry, and so they lump all those feelings together as signifying hunger, which leads them to overeat whenever they feel upset."

– Daniel Goleman, Ph.D.

Eat Your Heart Out

Hungry for love. Feeding the soul. Feeling empty inside. Have you ever noticed how many "eating" words are used to describe emotional states? There is a deeply intuitive connection between how hungry (or full) we are physically and how needy (or comfortable) we feel psychologically.

The connection is more than verbal. Our feelings often translate into certain eating behaviors. It seems like a simple goal to eat when we're hungry, to not eat when we're full, and to not eat for other reasons. But many people find it difficult to know when they're physically hungry and when they're eating for other reasons.

If you've established a life-long habit of eating in response to emotional cues, this can be a difficult pattern to change. There is no magic formula for changing this pattern, except learning to identify when you're physically hungry and responding appropriately by eating, and to recognize when you are emotionally uncomfortable and responding to those signals by doing something *instead of* eating.

Anger is often a trigger for overeating. You could argue that there's no logical connection between being angry and putting food in your mouth. But when you stop and think about it, you'll realize that there's a very direct connection. Putting food in your mouth when you're angry has the effect of dulling that feeling. Instead of getting expressed, your anger gets repressed and stuffed down inside. In this sense, eating "works." You get to feel angry with no risk, conflict, or consequences. What ultimately happens, of course, is that you end up carrying around a lot of unexpressed rage in a body that grows bigger and more burdened with every unexpressed conflict.

See if you can begin today to distinguish physical hunger from emotional hunger. And when you determine that your need to eat is purely from feelings, try helping yourself feel better in some other way.

EAT BETTER: The Benefits of Vitamin E

Postmenopausal women who eat foods rich in vitamin E lower their risk of death from heart disease. A University of Minnesota study has found that women with the highest intake of vitamin E had less than half the risk of death from coronary heart disease compared to women with the lowest intake of vitamin E.

Their vitamin E came from food rather than from supplements. Which foods are high in vitamin E? Wheat germ, avocados, sunflower seeds, nuts (especially almonds and filberts), vegetable oils, margarine, and mayonnaise. These foods can be high in fat, so as always, think in terms of moderation.

MOVE MORE: Kitchen Kapers

In the spirit of our commitment to move more during the course of daily life, we hereby offer you some fun ideas for benefiting your body while you're cooking, talking on the phone, or watching TV.

SOUP CAN TRICEPS TONER

1. Hold a can of soup (or beans, or tomato sauce. . . you get the idea) in your right hand as a weight.

2. Hold the can behind your head, palm facing forward.

3. Keep your upper arm stationary, exhale, and raise the can upward toward the ceiling.

4. Repeat this arm extender twenty times and then switch arms.

SOUP CAN OPENERS

1. Stand with your feet shoulder-width apart and parallel.

2. Grasp a soup can in each hand and extend your arms straight in front of you at chest level.

3. Slowly open your arms to the side, as you exhale.

4. Close them to the original position, as you inhale.

5. Repeat twelve times.

6. You can add knee bends as a variation. Slowly bend your knees as you open your arms.

DAZZLING DISH LEGS

1. While you are standing at the sink doing dishes or peeling potatoes, slowly raise your right leg to the side and hold it for ten seconds.

2. Repeat ten times and then switch legs.

3. To pick up the pace, hold each leg lift for one second instead of ten seconds.

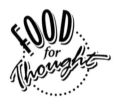

"Act as if it were impossible to fail."

— Dorothea Brande

STRESS LESS: A Nice Thing

Today, do one nice and unexpected thing for someone without anticipating or expecting anything in return. Bring a co-worker a cup of coffee, go out of your way to hold the door for someone struggling with packages, compliment the person on the phone who has helped you, offer to find those lost keys, let that older person take your place in line. What can you add to the list?

DAILY ACTION PLAN

Week _____   Day _____

Date _____   Weight _____

Breakfast	Time:	Protein Grams	Fat Grams	Carbs Grams	Calories
Protein:					
Fruit:					
Grain:					
Beverage:					
Snack	Time:				
Lunch	Time:				
Protein:					
Vegetable:					
Lettuce:					
Grain:					
Fruit:					
Miscellaneous:					
Beverage:					
Snack	Time:				
Dinner	Time:				
Protein:					
Vegetable:					
Lettuce:					
Grain:					
Fruit:					
Miscellaneous:					
Beverage:					
Snack	Time:				
TOTAL					

Today I was able to *Eat Better* by...

_____

_____

_____

_____

Today I was able to *Move More* by...

_____

_____

_____

Today I was able to *Stress Less* by...

_____

_____

_____

_____

_____

Today I feel really great about...

_____

_____

_____

_____

Tomorrow I will focus on...

_____

_____

_____

_____

DAY 19

"Through your actions, you can create conditions that change your brain chemistry, and therefore change your mental state, in ways that can make it easier for you to accomplish a specific purpose, such as achieving and maintaining lean weight."

– *Cynthia Stamper Graff*

What to Do Instead

I recently asked one of our successful Lean for Life maintainers if there were ever times when he experienced cravings but wasn't experiencing what he knew to be true hunger. He said there were. "What," I asked, "do you do when that happens?" He didn't hesitate to reply: "I do something else," he said matter-of-factly.

His answer was short and to the point. What do you do when you feel like eating but have decided not to? There are many reasons for deciding not to eat. You may realize you're not really hungry but are reaching for food out of habit. You may be experiencing an emotional craving and decide you don't want to give in to it. You may want to wait a little longer because your lunch date is picking you up in half an hour. You may have decided to "save" some calories for later.

Take a moment to think of what you've done in the past to distract yourself. An informal survey in our office yielded these suggestions:

- I walk down to get the mail.

- I drink another glass of water.

- I do some stretching exercises.

- I do a mental relaxation exercise.

- I listen to my favorite tape on my stereo headset.

- I play with the dog.

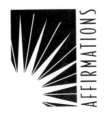

AFFIRMATIONS

"I can change my relationship with food."

- I take a short nap.

- I get up and move around and that seems to shake me up.

- I become engrossed in a project.

- I tell myself that if I still want it in 20 minutes, I'll eat it then.

All of these people said they had the experience of the hunger passing. If it doesn't, they at least make a more conscious, deliberate choice about what to eat. So think about ways you can respond next time you find yourself reaching for food you don't necessarily need or want. That way, you'll be prepared when it happens.

EAT BETTER: Salad Dressing

According to *Environmental Nutrition: The Newsletter of Food, Nutrition, and Health*, four tablespoons of the typical restaurant salad dressing can easily add up to 700 calories and 50 grams of fat to your salad. Is it worth it? Ask for dressing on the side. Dip your fork into it before bites rather than pouring it over the salad. You'll be surprised how much you leave behind.

When you're at home and can make your own dressing, you have more choices. Here are some suggestions for low fat dressing:

- Add seasonings to low fat yogurt or blended tofu.

- Use seasoned rice wine vinegar without any oil at all.

- Substitute chicken or vegetable stock for some or all of the oil in a vinaigrette.

- Substitute V-8 or tomato juice for some or all of the oil in a vinaigrette.

- Add seasonings to low-sodium soy sauce.

- Add seasonings to your favorite commercial low fat dressing. (Adding a little lemon juice will freshen up commercial dressings.)

- Add seasonings to a nonfat or low fat mayonnaise.

Many of our most successful Lean for Life maintainers take homemade dressing with them to restaurants. You can also find some tasty commercial nonfat or low fat dressing in the gourmet section of your grocery store. Shop carefully, read labels, and enjoy.

 ## MOVE MORE: Put On Your Dancing Shoes

How can something so much fun be so good for you? Dancing is one of the best forms of exercise. If you've ever watched a ballroom dance competition on TV or gone to the ballet, you know what effect dancing has on the body. Dancing combines two of the most powerful mood enhancers–music and body movement.

Just for fun, plan to dance your heart out for 30 minutes at least once this week. You can make a dance date with a friend, a child, or your partner. Or you can make a date with yourself. You can groove to the music and make up the moves as you go, or you can develop a routine.

Here's a suggestion. Choose music that is upbeat and has a good rhythm. My favorites are the Temptations and the Four Tops. Starting with your right foot, step to the right, and bring your left foot together with the right. Shift your weight to your left foot and step right again. Then kick your left foot. Then reverse the sequence, stepping to the left. Repeat this set eight times. Then do a variation. Starting with your right foot, step right and kick your left foot out. Then step left and kick your right foot out. Repeat this set eight times.

It sounds more complicated than it is. Here's a simple summary:

1. Right-together-right-kick.

2. Left-together-left-kick.

3. Repeat eight times.

4. Right-kick and left-kick.

5. Repeat eight times.

After you've mastered this "sophisticated" choreography, make up your own. It doesn't matter what steps you use. What matters is that you move!

DAILY ACTION PLAN

Week _____   Day _____

Date _____   Weight _____

Breakfast	Time:		Protein Grams	Fat Grams	Carbs Grams	Calories
Protein:						
Fruit:						
Grain:						
Beverage:						
Snack	Time:					
Lunch	Time:					
Protein:						
Vegetable:						
Lettuce:						
Grain:						
Fruit:						
Miscellaneous:						
Beverage:						
Snack	Time:					
Dinner	Time:					
Protein:						
Vegetable:						
Lettuce:						
Grain:						
Fruit:						
Miscellaneous:						
Beverage:						
Snack	Time:					
TOTAL						

Today I was able to *Eat Better* by...

_____
_____
_____
_____

Today I was able to *Move More* by...

_____
_____
_____

Today I was able to *Stress Less* by...

_____
_____
_____
_____

Today I feel really great about...

_____
_____
_____

Tomorrow I will focus on...

_____
_____
_____

STRESS LESS: The Spiritual Side of Life

There's clearly more to life than we can verify with our own senses. There are significant experiences that can't be observed or recreated, and that leave no physical evidence, even though people will tell you they are among the most important, empowering experiences they've ever had. Without them life would be dull and void of meaning.

Have you ever thrilled to the words of a song or a poem? Have you found your feelings perfectly expressed in a piece of music, even though you couldn't put them into words? Do you remember what it's like to look up at the night sky and see a glittering canopy of stars overhead? Have you ever felt truly forgiven? Or redeemed? Or loved?

These matters of the spirit are often private, but they are essential. What are you doing today to nourish your own spiritual life? Perhaps you are reminded of the truth and power of what cannot be seen when you go to church or stand in a forest or at the edge of the ocean. Maybe you find it when you look into your child's face. Or maybe, like Mother Teresa, you find it in the desperately poor and sick people of the streets. Be open to it. It's everywhere.

DAY 20

"It's entirely up to you how much you want to improve your health and whether you want to eat for yourself or to suit the convenience of restaurant owners, airline stewardesses, and the neighbors."

– Nathan Pritikin

Going Out to Eat

If you've decided you want to cut the fat in your diet and watch your calories, you can take heart in knowing you're in good company. At any given time, at least half the adults in this country are trying to lose weight.

Because you're not alone in your quest to eat better, you'll find it easier than ever to ask questions and make requests in restaurants without feeling like an alien. Asking whether the steamed vegetables are buttered or whether the fish is broiled or fried is perfectly acceptable, as well as an intelligent thing to do.

Besides gathering information, you can even take it a step further and make requests. Once you become knowledgeable about how much fat there is in a pat of butter or the dressing on your salad, you can decide for yourself whether it's worth it. You can ask them to hold the mayo or ask for your omelette without cheese.

In addition, many restaurants are adding "heart healthy" dishes that are low in calories and fat grams. They have learned that such choices make patrons happy and actually increases their business. Even fast food places offer plain baked potatoes, low fat bean burritos, or nonfat muffins.

The bottom line is that it's easier than ever to walk into any restaurant and make healthful choices. They're already available, or at least available for the asking. They key is you. Are you committed enough to take advantage of your options?

EAT BETTER: Drinking Green Tea

For some time now, human and animal studies have been finding a link between tea and good health. Green tea has substantial health benefits. It's made from the unfermented leaves of the tea plant. Black tea is made from the same plant, but the leaves are fermented. In the process of fermentation, certain compounds called catechins are mostly destroyed, thus making black tea healthful, but not as healthful as green tea.

The catechins in green tea lower blood levels of LDL, the "bad" cholesterol, and increase levels of HDL, the "good" cholesterol. Green tea also reduces the risk of stomach cancer, and possibly other cancers. And it reduces the risk of stroke.

However, the antioxidant properties of green tea seem to be destroyed if you add milk to your tea. Milk proteins apparently bind with catechins to make them unavailable. The more milk you add, the less able green tea is to do its unique work on behalf of your health. Recent research has found comparable benefits to drinking black tea. So have a tea party and enjoy!

MOVE MORE: The Sit Down Workout

Most of us spend an awful lot of time sitting down. When we don't move, we get stiff and weak. We also tend to get tired. Here are some simple sitting exercises that will help keep you flexible and energized.

ARM CIRCLES

1. Stretch your arms out to the sides, shoulder high.

2. With palms up, make small backward circles in the air.

3. Start with ten repetitions and increase as time and energy permit.

WAIST WHITTLER

1. Sit tall, stretch your arms over your head and interlock your thumbs.

2. Keeping your arms straight, bend at the waist so you lean first to the right and then to the left.

3. Repeat five times.

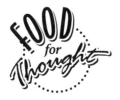

SIT DOWN STRETCHES

1. Sit tall and stretch your arms straight overhead.

2. Bend at the waist and touch the ground.

3. Do ten repetitions.

CHAIR JOGGING

1. Sit tall in your chair and hold on to the edge of your chair for support.

2. Lift your legs so you are jogging in place as fast as you can.

3. Continue for two minutes.

HIGH KICKS

1. Sit tall in your chair and hold onto the chair for support.

2. Straighten one leg and lift as high off the ground as you can.

3. Return to starting position.

4. Repeat with the other leg.

5. Do ten repetitions.

FOOT FLEX

1. Sit tall in your chair and hold on to the edge for support.

2. Straighten one leg and raise it off the ground.

3. Flex and point your foot so that your toes are aligned with your leg. Repeat eight times.

4. Repeat with the other leg.

STRESS LESS: Recovering from Stressful Events

There are many things you can do to help yourself recover from stressful situations. First, you can resume your regular, healthful habits. Eat well, start exercising again, get enough sleep, and reach out to other people to love and be loved.

DAILY ACTION PLAN

Week _____   Day _____

Date _____   Weight _____

Breakfast	Time:	Protein Grams	Fat Grams	Carbs Grams	Calories
Protein:					
Fruit:					
Grain:					
Beverage:					
Snack	Time:				
Lunch	Time:				
Protein:					
Vegetable:					
Lettuce:					
Grain:					
Fruit:					
Miscellaneous:					
Beverage:					
Snack	Time:				
Dinner	Time:				
Protein:					
Vegetable:					
Lettuce:					
Grain:					
Fruit:					
Miscellaneous:					
Beverage:					
Snack	Time:				
TOTAL					

Today I was able to *Eat Better* by...

_____
_____
_____
_____

Today I was able to *Move More* by...

_____
_____
_____

Today I was able to *Stress Less* by...

_____
_____
_____
_____

Today I feel really great about...

_____
_____
_____
_____

Tomorrow I will focus on...

_____
_____
_____
_____

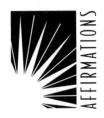

AFFIRMATIONS

"I feel good about choosing foods that nourish me and keep me healthy."

In addition, you can start practicing relaxation/visualization techniques twice a day. Deep breathing, progressive muscle relaxation, mental imaging, and meditation help your body return to a more normal, healthy state after intense or prolonged stress.

How you *think* about what happens to you is just as important as what actually happens. Pay attention to the words you use to tell yourself the story of your life. Consciously choose to interpret events so that you're as optimistic as possible, interrupt self-destructive thoughts, and banish negative images. Pay attention to the specifics of your situation so you don't make the mistake of generalizing your distress.

You may need to talk out your feelings and explore them in some depth with someone you trust. And, depending on the difficulty, you may need to be patient with yourself. We've all heard that time is the greatest healer of all. Living that truth can require faith and loving patience.

Alcohol and Estrogen

A recent study at Brigham and Women's Hospital in Boston looked at the effects that drinking alcohol has on blood levels of estradiol, the body's major form of estrogen. The study found that alcohol increases estrogen levels significantly in women who have completed menopause and who are taking oral estrogen.

The excessive estrogen circulating in the blood may promote breast cancer. In fact, women on estrogen who consume as little as 1 1/2 to 2 alcoholic beverages a day may be exposed to unhealthful estrogen levels. Although occasional social drinkers have no cause to worry, women on hormone replacement therapy who regularly consume alcohol should discuss their concerns with their doctors.

DAY 21

"When you walk in the door from work on a busy day there is an in-between time, a string of moments when you don't know what to do with yourself, so you open the refrigerator. You want to eat, it would taste good, but you're not hungry. And you can't think of anything to do that sounds as good as eating. That's the moment where the choice has to be made. Again."

– Geneen Roth

Cravings

You know how food cravings can be. They're cunning and merciless. They emerge from nowhere to eclipse our self-control and derail our best intentions. And when it happens, you feel powerless and doomed.

Or are you? Food cravings aren't really mysterious urges sent from the underworld to torment and distract you. Cravings are complex, but they can be understood and they can be neutralized.

You can understand more than you do now by carefully observing your own craving patterns. Once you see what's happening, you can take intentional action to intervene in positive ways. Here are some questions to ask yourself:

- Are you experiencing a craving because you've allowed yourself get too hungry? If so, you can get back on track by establishing a predictable eating schedule that allows you to feel satisfied.

- Are you experiencing a craving because you're having a conditioned response to something in your external environment? Do you drink too much on New Year's Eve? Do do eat buttered popcorn at the movies? Do you overeat every time you walk up to an all-you-can-eat buffet or salad bar? If so, you can teach yourself to have a different response to "danger zones" that have caused you to overindulge in the past.

- Are you experiencing cravings because you aren't physically active enough? If so, you know you can control your appetite by consistently engaging in moderate exercise every day.

- Are you experiencing a craving because you're feeling emotions you don't know how to deal with? If so, you can express how you're really feeling to yourself or someone else. You can feel the feeling and lose the fear.

- Are you experiencing a craving because you're just too tired? If so, you can take a nap or do a relaxation or visualization session.

- Are you experiencing a craving because you're premenstrual? If so, you might want to have an extra healthy snack or two during the day.

We all experience occasional cravings, but they don't have to possess or control us. We can be aware of why we're experiencing them, consider what happens when we give in, practice delaying our gratification, engage in alternative activities, and give ourselves credit for becoming a stronger person–mentally, emotionally, and physically.

EAT BETTER: Food Diary Check-In

You're now at the end of your third week of the program. This is a perfect time to pause and take a look at how you're eating. You've been filling out your Daily Action Plan every day, so you now have 21 days of information regarding on your eating habits. That's more than enough data to reveal patterns and identify problems.

Let's review. Take your time to answer the questions below, and refer to your Daily Action Plan forms when you need to.

- Calculate the average number of calories you're eating for each week. Are you staying within the calorie limit that you set for yourself?

- Calculate the average number of fat grams you're eating each week. Are you staying within the 30% limit?

- Do you feel that your appetite is within balance? Are you too hungry or too full?

DAILY ACTION PLAN

Week _____   Day _____

Date _____   Weight _____

Breakfast Time:	Protein Grams	Fat Grams	Carbs Grams	Calories
Protein:				
Fruit:				
Grain:				
Beverage:				
Snack Time:				
Lunch Time:				
Protein:				
Vegetable:				
Lettuce:				
Grain:				
Fruit:				
Miscellaneous:				
Beverage:				
Snack Time:				
Dinner Time:				
Protein:				
Vegetable:				
Lettuce:				
Grain:				
Fruit:				
Miscellaneous:				
Beverage:				
Snack Time:				
TOTAL				

Today I was able to *Eat Better* by...

_____

_____

_____

_____

Today I was able to *Move More* by...

_____

_____

_____

Today I was able to *Stress Less* by...

_____

_____

_____

_____

Today I feel really great about...

_____

_____

_____

_____

Tomorrow I will focus on...

_____

_____

_____

_____

- Are you enjoying your food? Are there enough "treats" during the week to satisfy you? Are you feeling deprived?

- Are you eating a healthy diet? Are there foods you want to be eating more often? Less often?

If you've answered "No" to any of these questions, you can greet this information with open arms. Now is the time to be sensitive to problems and do what you can to correct them. Everyone has to make adjustments as they go along, and reviewing your eating patterns every so often is a convenient way to keep small problems from becoming overwhelming.

MOVE MORE: How Are You Moving?

This is also a great time to review your level of physical activity. You've been keeping track of your exercise and everyday activities in your Daily Action Plan. What patterns do you notice? What can you learn about yourself from the records you've been keeping over the past three weeks?

- Are you engaging in intentional activity several times a week?

- Is your level of activity staying the same, decreasing, or increasing?

- Are you getting a variety of activity, or do you focus primarily on one thing?

- What would you like to see yourself doing differently for the next five weeks?

- What is one activity goal that you can identify for the coming week?

An occasional review of these questions will help you stay focused and keep your physical activity fresh, challenging, and effective throughout your life.

STRESS LESS: Be Like Mother Nature

Study after study has demonstrated that people who have living things to care for are less stressed and happier than those who don't (unless, of course, those living things are teenagers, and then all bets are off!).

Perhaps the easiest, cheapest, and most secure investment you can make in this regard is to care for a plant. If you mess up, the consequences are relatively minor compared to what happens when you make mistakes with children or pets.

Sometime in the next few days, find yourself a plant to care for. Depending on the season, you can plant something outdoors in a container or in the ground. If, on the other hand, you are reading this in the middle of a snow storm, you can find an indoor plant to remind you that things change. The sharp-edged cold of winter always softens into the vibrant warmth of spring.

You can play a small part in the mysterious and beautiful cycle of life that allows tender green shoots to emerge from hard, black seeds, and soft pink blossoms to flower from sticks.

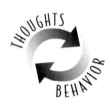

MENTAL FITNESS: Controlling Cravings

You know how it usually goes when you have a craving for something. Your interest becomes a preoccupation, which soon mushrooms into an obsession. And when you indulge yourself, you follow a well-worn trail that inevitably leads to hopelessness:

FOOD THOUGHT OR CRAVING → GIVE IN → EAT → FEEL GUILTY → GIVE UP

This may feel inevitable and you may feel out of control. But it *is* not, and you *are* not. It is possible to interrupt this sequence and change it. Then the sequence looks more like this:

FOOD THOUGHT OR CRAVING → STOP! → TAKE A DEEP BREATH →

OBSERVE → PLAN OF ACTION

Let's take a closer look at what this means. Whenever you are tempted to do anything that might interfere with your program, STOP!

STOP! Visualize a stop sign and hear the word "stop." Immediately stop what you are doing.

TAKE three deep cleansing breaths. This interrupts the physical and emotional sequence that has lead to guilt and defeat in the past. You now have an opportunity to do things differently.

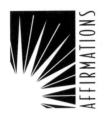

AFFIRMATIONS

"I am in charge of
what I eat,
when I eat, and
how much I eat."

OBSERVE yourself. How do you feel? What do you want? What really matters to you? What choices do you have?

PLAN a course of action. Sometimes you really need to eat something. If you do, make your food choice in a conscious and controlled way. But often your hunger is not really for food; you are looking for something else. Make a conscious choice to meet the real need. Take a walk. Sit quietly for five or ten minutes. Read something. Take a bath. Call a friend. Listen to music. Work on a creative project.

Through this process, you'll learn that you can meet your needs in ways that are good for you. You'll broaden your options instead of having just one way to respond to anger, sadness, fear, loneliness, excitement, joy, and the many other emotions you're capable of feeling.

Your Turn. Living With Gratitude

Today I live my life with an attitude of gratitude.

Today I am grateful for_____

_____

_____

_____

_____

_____

_____

_____

_____

_____

_____

WEEK 4

MOVEMENT: The Beauty of a Well-Used Body

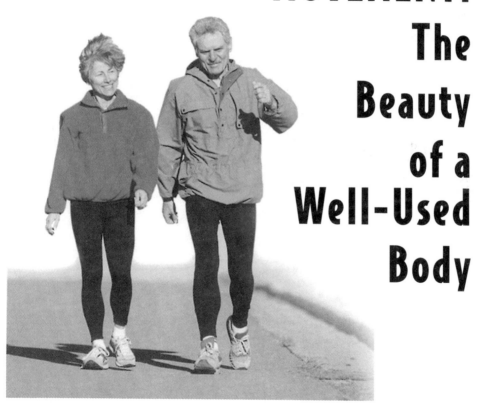

How you feel about your body, and how your care for it, are important factors in your maintenance program. You can learn to appreciate your body for the intricate and beautiful way it works, and you can stretch your own limits by becoming physically active.

DAY 22

"A middle-aged client was complaining of his daily fatigue. His work exhausted him, and every day when he returned home he was fragmented. 'The only thing which helps me,' he said, 'is when I climb up the mountain right near my house.' It was a modest mountain, really just a large hill, which he could hike up and back down in about an hour. 'Then why don't you climb it every day?' I asked."

– John A. Sanford

Then Why Don't You Climb It?

Sometimes the simplest, most obvious action makes the most sense. Instead of getting your ideas of what you *ought* to be doing from reading or talking with other people, trust your instincts and ask yourself what *you* want to do.

If you're thinking of putting together an exercise program, ask yourself what kind of physical activity makes you feel good. What do you enjoy? What activities did you enjoy as a child or adolescent? What looks like fun? Let yourself be guided by your answer.

I know a woman who talked wistfully about how the wind flowed through her hair when she rode her bike as a kid. She loved it. She dreamed about it. But for some reason, it never occurred to her that riding a bicycle would be a wonderful form of exercise today. Somehow, she hadn't considered her own enjoyment to be important. She equated exercise with hard work.

Pay attention to what you love. If you're not sure what that is, give yourself the opportunity to try a number of possibilities. Maybe you'll love the individual challenge of rock climbing, or the artistic expression of dance, or the team spirit of doubles tennis. Maybe you like the meditative aspects of walking alone, or the camaraderie of aerobics.

The best part of doing what you like to do is you'll enjoy doing it!

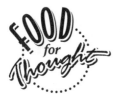

EAT BETTER: Serving Sizes

Many of us use a kitchen scale and measuring cups at home to zero in on accurate serving portions. But what about when you're eating away from home? You can't very well take out your cup measure in a nice restaurant and spoon your pasta into it. But you can do a pretty good job of estimating how much you're about to eat. Here are some tips.

PASTA OR RICE
A half cup serving of pasta or rice is about the size of the palm of your hand.

FRUIT
A medium apple, pear, peach, or other fruit is about the size of your fist when your thumb is held up toward you. That's about 2" square. A medium banana is about 5" long.

MEAT OR FISH
A serving size of meat is about the size of a deck of playing cards. A serving size of fish is slightly larger.

A good way to perfect your estimates is to regularly measure your food at home. Before long, you'll get used to accurately estimating serving sizes.

MOVE MORE: Walking, the Magic Pill

For the first time in American history, more than half of all Americans are overweight. Not only is all that excess weight hard on our bodies, it's a drain on our national pocketbook. According to a Brown University study, if every sedentary American walked an hour a day, we would not only slim down, but we'd save $20 billion in health care costs every year.

STRESS LESS: A Visualization of Yourself as a Beloved Child

We have such high expectations for ourselves. So many of us get caught up in doing more, having more, and being better. There's nothing wrong with aiming high, but there

DAILY ACTION PLAN

Week _____ Day _____

Date _____ Weight _____

Breakfast Time:	Protein Grams	Fat Grams	Carbs Grams	Calories
Protein:				
Fruit:				
Grain:				
Beverage:				
Snack Time:				
Lunch Time:				
Protein:				
Vegetable:				
Lettuce:				
Grain:				
Fruit:				
Miscellaneous:				
Beverage:				
Snack Time:				
Dinner Time:				
Protein:				
Vegetable:				
Lettuce:				
Grain:				
Fruit:				
Miscellaneous:				
Beverage:				
Snack Time:				
TOTAL				

Today I was able to *Eat Better* by...

_____
_____
_____
_____

Today I was able to *Move More* by...

_____
_____
_____
_____

Today I was able to *Stress Less* by...

_____
_____
_____
_____
_____
_____

Today I feel really great about...

_____
_____
_____
_____

Tomorrow I will focus on...

_____
_____
_____
_____
_____

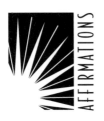

AFFIRMATIONS

"I enjoy living a healthy life every day."

is something destructive about being overly hard on ourselves. Along with our desire for self-improvement, there must come an increasing acceptance of our own quirks, imperfections, and limitations.

There is a way to craft a more tolerant and less judgmental stance with regard to our own performance. We can learn to treat ourselves as gently as we would treat a beloved child. And we can get in touch with ourselves as a beloved child by practicing this visualization.

Close your eyes and take three long, relaxing, deep breaths. Let yourself be in a safe room from your childhood, perhaps your own bedroom. Look around you and notice what it looks like and what it sounds like. Let yourself experience the safety you feel in that place. Become aware of the presence of someone who loved you as a child–maybe a parent, grandparent, or teacher. You can see this person's face and the way he or she is smiling at you. You know that this adult loves and cherishes you. What do you think this person is communicating to you? Take a few minutes to become aware of the feelings this person has for the child you once were.

After this visualization session is over, continue to think about the feelings that were generated when you were able to put yourself back into a safe place with a trusted adult. How can you carry these feelings with you into your daily activities?

SUCCESS STORY: Mark Huckenpahler

At 46, Mark Huckenpahler is the picture of good health. Strong and lean, he stands 5'7", weighs 142 pounds, and looks like a world-class athlete who knows–and enjoys–the benefits of fitness.

But there was a time just eight years ago when Mark was a world-class couch potato. He weighed 212 pounds, avoided mirrors, and had a tough time walking because of severe knee pain resulting from years of being overweight.

"I felt like a real pile of crap," he remembers. "I hated the way I looked. I was a slob. I avoided people and basically ate, slept, watched television, and did odd jobs to get by. I feel like a totally different human being today. My life has totally changed."

Indeed it has. The day he began his Lean for Life program, he landed a job with a major home improvement retailer, a position he still holds. He also began running when a neighbor encouraged him to enter a local 5K race, and hasn't stopped since. Over the past six years, Mark has completed 130 running events, including 20 marathons!

Two years ago, Mark decided to pursue a goal that only a handful of people in the world have ever accomplished: to run marathons on all seven continents. He completed marathons in North America, South America, Asia, Antarctica, Africa and Europe. On January 1, 2000, Mark achieved his dream when he completed the Millennium Marathon in New Zealand.

"When people ask me why I run so much, the answer is easy: because I can," says Mark. "There was a time when tying my shoes and walking out to my car caused me to break a sweat. I was a fat kid, and I know how difficult it is to move around and to feel good about yourself when you're overweight. I'm thankful every day that I finally did something about it and have the ability to move and use my body the way I do today."

Mark says his level of activity isn't the only change he's maintained since achieving his weight loss goal.

"I used to eat for pleasure," he explains. "Now I eat for fuel. I'm much more aware of what my body wants and needs to operate at maximum efficiency. Every time I eat, I ask myself, 'What will this food do *for* me–or *to* me?'

Mark runs six miles, two or three days a week, and varies his training schedule with kayaking and weight training at a local gym.

"As healthy and fit as I feel today, I never forget what it felt like to be fat," says Mark. "When I was overweight, I had no idea how much life I was missing out on. That's something I'll never allow to happen again. I'm making up for lost time, and I'm having the time of my life doing it."

DAY 23

"There is a magic in skiing when all is going well which transcends anything I have experienced in other sports. As I soar down a mountainside letting my body find its own balance in turn after turn, my mind as clear as the cold air against my face, my heart feels as warm as the sun, and I attain a level of experience which compels me to return to the snow for more and more of the same."
– Timothy Gallwey and Bob Kriegel

Step It Up for Greater Results!

At Lindora, one of our very favorite tools for weight loss and maintenance is the pedometer. When you walk down the halls of our corporate office, you're likely to see these small plastic devices clipped to belts, peeking out under jackets, and even attached to shoes. They are everywhere, and for good reason: they're designed to monitor and measure your level of activity.

When we first started wearing them, none of us had a truly accurate, objective measurement of how active we really were. In the same way that people tend to underestimate their calories, they tend to overestimate their activity level and the number of steps they take every day. So, right from the start, the pedometer proved itself indispensable. It gives you an accurate record of your steps. You can't fudge. If the counter says 4,786 steps, then it's 4,786 steps. There's no room for denial.

We soon found the pedometer helpful in other ways. Not only was it a "recorder," but it was also a fabulous "cheerleader." Most of us found ourselves checking our pedometers periodically during the day just to see how we were doing. It was a benign but persistent reminder of our commitment to be active.

Sometimes, you'll steal a quick look and smile because you've taken more steps than you thought. Other times, you think to yourself that you'd better "step it up" by the end of the day or you'll never hit your 10,000 step goal. It's not uncommon to see people at our office happily marching in place while on the telephone, glancing every so often at a small white cube clipped to their waist.

Remember: When you increase your activity level, you improve your overall health. So step it up!

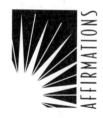

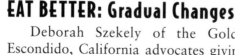

EAT BETTER: Gradual Changes

Deborah Szekely of the Golden Door Spa in Escondido, California advocates giving up one fattening food each decade. She reasons that since we generally tend to burn fewer calories as we age and it becomes easier to put on weight, we need to make a conscious choice to counterbalance these changes.

Imagine the cumulative difference it would have made if you had given up butter in your twenties, peanut butter in your thirties, cheddar cheese in your forties, cream in your coffee in your fifties, and chocolate in your sixties. Of course, we don't really mean "give up" as in give up in the same way that an alcoholic would do well to give up alcohol. We mean that these foods become occasional treats rather than every day staples.

Gradual, cumulative changes add up to big differences over time. No matter how old you are right now, consider how you might make use of this idea.

MOVE MORE: Sedentary Habits Increase Risk of Heart Disease

Men and women who are unfit are seven to eight times more likely to have cardiovascular disease than those who are fit. In effect, this means that the more physically active you are, the less likely you are to have heart disease. In other words, regular physical activity helps protect against heart attacks.

Approximately 20 - 25% of the adult population is not active and not fit, and therefore at high risk. That's 40 million Americans. These numbers give a sense of urgency to strategies that get people up and moving.

Adding an intentional period of exercise during the day is one effective way to increase physical activity. So is looking for opportunities to use up energy during the course of your normal day. How you do it isn't as important as finding ways to be active every day. It's up to you. You can take charge of your own activity level, keep track of your

"It feels good to move my body."

progress, and find ways to move through the obstacles. You'll do a better job of solving the problems than some expert who doesn't know you, isn't living your life, and wouldn't necessarily understand what activities are feasible for you to do regularly.

STRESS LESS: The Joy of the Journal

There is all kinds of evidence from all kinds of studies that keeping a journal will help you cope better with difficulties and stay physically healthy. Writing about your feelings for 20 minutes a day actually boosts the number of cells in your body that attack viruses and bacteria.

Likewise, a food diary will help you stay in control of your eating, solve problems, and get to know yourself better. Many highly creative people (artists, writers, musicians) keep journals for the purpose of capturing insights and exploring ideas that would otherwise never come fully to their conscious attention. Other people keep journals as a way of strengthening a sense of identity and expressing feelings safely.

We encourage people on the Lean for Life program to keep a journal. Many of the topics introduced in this book lend themselves to further exploration through writing. If you would like to keep a journal, here are some suggestions:

- Buy a notebook or journal that invites you and doesn't intimidate you. You don't want to feel that every word is inscribed for posterity. You want to feel comfortable.

- Understand from the beginning that the benefit is in the process of writing more than it is in the finished product. You want to be free to express yourself fully without worrying about the quality of the writing.

- Establish privacy for yourself. A journal that is kept with any concern that someone else may read it will be half-hearted and half-truthful. A journal is a record of feelings "of the moment" rather than a record of the truth for all time.

- Regular writing sessions establish the journaling habit. But whether that means writing at the same time, same place every day, or several times a week as the spirit moves, is up to you.

DAILY ACTION PLAN

Week _____   Day _____

Date _____   Weight _____

Breakfast Time:	Protein Grams	Fat Grams	Carbs Grams	Calories
Protein:				
Fruit:				
Grain:				
Beverage:				
Snack Time:				
Lunch Time:				
Protein:				
Vegetable:				
Lettuce:				
Grain:				
Fruit:				
Miscellaneous:				
Beverage:				
Snack Time:				
Dinner Time:				
Protein:				
Vegetable:				
Lettuce:				
Grain:				
Fruit:				
Miscellaneous:				
Beverage:				
Snack Time:				
TOTAL				

Today I was able to *Eat Better* by...

_____

_____

_____

_____

Today I was able to *Move More* by...

_____

_____

_____

Today I was able to *Stress Less* by...

_____

_____

_____

Today I feel really great about...

_____

_____

_____

Tomorrow I will focus on...

_____

_____

_____

_____

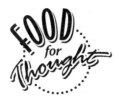

As an experiment, you could commit to keeping a journal for one month and then evaluate your experience. Was it valuable? Do you think it helps you move toward your goals? If the answer is yes, then you have the power of your own experience as encouragement to continue.

More Evidence in Favor of Fruits and Vegetables

It is possible to lower blood pressure through diet alone. The DASH study (Dietary Approaches to Stopping Hypertension) found that eating a diet that is loaded with fruits and vegetables (9 to 10 servings a day) can decrease blood pressure within two weeks. The decrease is equivalent to treatment with drugs.

Researchers speculate that the abundance of potassium, magnesium, calcium, fiber and other nutrients are responsible for the healthful effects. As is often the case, however, getting these nutrients from food seems to be more effective than taking supplements for any one nutrient.

"While all humans may be preprogrammed to walk, for example, there is much evidence that we are not all born dancers or hockey players or violinists. Somehow, though, we learn how to do all manner of things, from tying a shoe to driving a car, which then become second nature."
— The editors of Time Life Books

Mitochrondria 101

Between 70% to 90% of the calories you burn each day get burned in your muscle cells. If you are in balance, by the end of the day you will have burned as much fat as you have stored. Or, if you are in the process of losing excess fat, you will have burned more fat than you have stored.

In order to burn fat for fuel, mitochrondria need to be present in your muscle cells. Too small to be seen with an ordinary microscope, these tiny, egg-shaped structures function as little fat-burning furnaces. The more mitochondrial surface you have in your cells, the more efficient your body will be at burning body fat.

If your body isn't very efficient at using body fat for fuel, then fat will tend to accumulate, and you'll feel hungry and grumpy. You need as much mitochondria as possible to burn calories from the food you eat, and to feel comfortable and not hungry.

So what if you were shortchanged at birth in the mitochondria department? Is there anything you can do? Absolutely. You can intentionally increase your mitochondria. Tomorrow, we'll tell you how.

EAT BETTER: Eating for Health

We know that cutting fat and cholesterol reduces the risk of heart disease and diabetes. But cutting fat isn't enough to stay healthy. You also have to eat a variety of nutrient-rich foods to keep from getting sick. Snacking on reduced-fat cookies, crackers, potato chips, or other foods isn't good enough. What you need to do is toss out the fat free snacks and reach for raw fruits and vegetables instead.

The current recommendation is five to nine servings of fruits and vegetables every day. The National Cancer Institute estimates that less than 80% of the population eat even five servings. You need to cut the fat and eat more natural, nutrient-rich foods in order to help your body work well.

Remember, maintenance means both stabilizing your weight and guarding your good health. After all, there's no point in being thin but unhealthy.

MOVE MORE: Warming Up

Whether you're an accomplished athlete or exercising for the first time in years, it's always a good idea to warm up before you exercise.

Before you begin these warm-ups, change into loose, comfortable clothing and wear good athletic shoes. Drink a tall glass of water, and keep more water handy so you don't get thirsty during your exercise session.

WALKING IN PLACE

An easy way to get your body moving is simply to walk in place for a few minutes. Be sure to stand tall and swing your arms smoothly and naturally. You can take small steps or big steps, depending on your fitness level.

SHOULDER SHRUG

Stand with your head held high, your head facing forward, and your arms loose. Raise both shoulders as high as you can toward your ears. Relax as you bring them down. And then repeat.

THE SLOW MARCH

Stand next to a high-backed chair, with your head held high and your shoulders relaxed. Hold onto the back of the chair for support with your right hand, and raise your left knee until your thigh is parallel to the floor. Lower your foot gently to the floor. Shift your weight and raise your right knee until your right thigh is parallel to the floor. Lower your foot gently to the floor. Repeat.

Once you've completed your warm-ups, you'll be ready to go!

DAILY ACTION PLAN

Week _____   Day _____

Date _____   Weight _____

Breakfast	Time:		Protein Grams	Fat Grams	Carbs Grams	Calories
Protein:						
Fruit:						
Grain:						
Beverage:						
Snack	Time:					
Lunch	Time:					
Protein:						
Vegetable:						
Lettuce:						
Grain:						
Fruit:						
Miscellaneous:						
Beverage:						
Snack	Time:					
Dinner	Time:					
Protein:						
Vegetable:						
Lettuce:						
Grain:						
Fruit:						
Miscellaneous:						
Beverage:						
Snack	Time:					
TOTAL						

Today I was able to *Eat Better* by...

_____

_____

_____

_____

Today I was able to *Move More* by...

_____

_____

_____

Today I was able to *Stress Less* by...

_____

_____

_____

_____

_____

Today I feel really great about...

_____

_____

_____

Tomorrow I will focus on...

_____

_____

_____

STRESS LESS: Tracking Your Achievements

It's so important to keep track of your achievements. We're not just talking about major achievements like landing a better job or completing a marathon. We're talking about the small steps that take us one-by-one in the right direction, the little things you might easily overlook if you weren't paying attention.

Here are some examples of the kind of achievements that are worth celebrating: Increasing your steps over the course of a week. Staying within your calorie limit on the day you went to your sister's wedding. Doing a relaxation visualization in your car before you drove home from work. Filling out your Daily Action Plan every day for two weeks.

As you can see, there are hundreds of possibilities and reasons for feeling good about yourself. Take a minute or two right now to write down five. Was that easy? If so, add five more. This is the kind of thing you could note every day when you fill out your Daily Action Plan or write about in your journal. After a short while, you'll start feeling better about yourself. And that's a terrific way to feel when you're doing maintenance.

DAY 25

"Unless the heart and muscles are stressed beyond the normal range of activity for a given individual, there is no stimulus for their efficiency or capacity to improve."
– Jack W. Rejeski and Elizabeth A. Kenney

Mitochondria 102

You probably won't be surprised by the solution to yesterday's question: What can you do to increase the number and size of mitochondria in your muscle cells?

You guessed it. Exercise. The physiology of exercise and mitochondria is well known. All we have to say here is that, in addition to all the other benefits, exercise also works on a cellular level to change your body composition so that you increase your capacity to burn body fat.

Another piece of great news is that the exercise doesn't need to be intense. It can be moderate. Moderate is fine, as long as you do something every day. For most people, a good initial goal is 30 minutes five or six days a week. And the best way to start out is by walking. If walking for 30 minutes is too much, then do less. If 30 minutes isn't enough to leave you feeling challenged, then do more.

Remember, you want to do everything you can to build your body into a healthy, fat-burning system. Boosting your level of mitochondria is a perfect step in that direction. At Lindora, we urge everyone to become a Mitochrondriac®!

EAT BETTER: Snacking

When we think about snacking, most of us zero in on chips and dip, cookies and cakes, pizza and beer, or ice cream with hot fudge. We tend to think of snacks as exempt foods, foods outside the limits of regular nutrition that seem to exist only for our pig-out pleasure.

We need to change that notion. When you are on a maintenance program, snacks are the same kind of good food you eat at meals, only you eat them in-between breakfast, lunch, and dinner.

The creation of low fat and nonfat baked goods and junk food has lulled lots of people into thinking that they can eat as many low fat cookies as they want. The trouble is that low fat cookies still have calories. And when you eat a low fat cookie, you are not eating a peach. In other words, you're getting too many calories and not enough vitamins and minerals.

Good snacks come from the same categories as good food: lean meats, whole grains, fruits, vegetables, and skim milk products. Not many people snack on broiled chicken breasts at 4:00 in the afternoon. But there's no reason not to.

 ## MOVE MORE: More About Warming Up

Stretching should be an important part of your daily routine. Whether you take a "stretch break" away from your computer or stretch as part of your pre-exercise warm-up, these exercises will keep you strong and supple. Always remember to be gentle. Listen to your body and relax into these stretches, rather than force your way into them.

EASY HIP STRETCH

Lie on your back with your knees bent and the soles of your feet together. Slowly push your knees to the floor, only as far as is comfortable. Hold for 30 seconds, and repeat five times.

PUSHING THE WALL

Stand about three feet away from a wall and extend your arms forward past your head so your hands are supporting your weight on the wall. With your feet pointing straight ahead, step forward with one foot and bend your knee. Keep your other foot back. Lean forward as far as you comfortably can, keeping your back heel on the floor. You should feel the stretch in your calf and Achilles tendon. Hold for ten seconds, then reverse legs.

CHEST STRETCH

Stand in a doorway. Bend your elbows and grab the door frame at shoulder height, with your palms facing away from you. Put one foot in front of the other and bend your knee. Slowly lean forward through the doorway and hold for ten seconds. Repeat with the other leg forward.

DAILY ACTION PLAN

Week _____   Day _____

Date _____   Weight _____

Breakfast	Time:	Protein Grams	Fat Grams	Carbs Grams	Calories
Protein:					
Fruit:					
Grain:					
Beverage:					
Snack	Time:				
Lunch	Time:				
Protein:					
Vegetable:					
Lettuce:					
Grain:					
Fruit:					
Miscellaneous:					
Beverage:					
Snack	Time:				
Dinner	Time:				
Protein:					
Vegetable:					
Lettuce:					
Grain:					
Fruit:					
Miscellaneous:					
Beverage:					
Snack	Time:				
TOTAL					

Today I was able to *Eat Better* by...

_____
_____
_____
_____

Today I was able to *Move More* by...

_____
_____
_____
_____

Today I was able to *Stress Less* by...

_____
_____
_____
_____

Today I feel really great about...

_____
_____
_____

Tomorrow I will focus on...

_____
_____
_____

STRESS LESS: An Encouraging Word

A lot more people think of themselves as shy than you would think. While we now know that most children grow out of shyness, beginning around the age of twelve, there are a lot of us who think of ourselves as quiet and reserved throughout our lives.

As you go through your daily routine today, let yourself be sensitive to those around you who are quiet and unobtrusive–the young girl in the elevator, the older man who waits on you at the counter. Go out of your way to say something pleasant and friendly. A few warm words can do a lot to help people feel more connected and more valuable. There's already plenty of rude and even uncivil behavior in our culture. See what you can do to bring back on old-fashioned sense of courtesy and good manners. Kindness is the ultimate stress reducer. It makes the giver *and* the receiver both feel better.

SUCCESS STORY: Jason Andrews

There was a time when walking to the refrigerator was Jason Andrews' idea of a workout. He tipped the scales at 379 pounds, wore size 56 pants, and was growing increasingly concerned about his health.

"I felt like I was committing slow suicide," Jason remembers, "but it was really difficult to get motivated and take the first step."

It took the death of actor John Candy to stir Andrews into action.

"He was a young, energetic, big guy just like me," says Jason, a 42-year-old airline reservation supervisor. "When I heard he died, it really hit me. I realized that if I didn't start taking care of myself and make some big changes, the odds were good that I wasn't that far behind him. It was time to take pride and take control."

And that he did. Jason began his Lean for Life program right before Thanksgiving, 1996, and just days into his weight-loss program, made a commitment to exercise.

"When I first started walking, it was tough," Jason remembers. "Several of the routes I walk in my neighborhood are pretty hilly, and there were times I was sure I'd never make it to the top. I remember how proud I was of myself a few months later when I ran up this one particular hill. It was a real turning point in the way I felt about my body and my ability to become and stay healthy."

These days, it takes a lot more than a hill to intimidate Jason. He walks four miles a day at least six days a week.

"My wife and I walk together every morning at 4:20," says Jason. "It's a great way to start the day together. I also do 400 stomach crunches every day, 200 push-ups every other day, and I recently completed my first 5K run."

Today, Jason Andrews' life looks and feels very different. The results speak for themselves: he has lost more than 165 pounds and 20 inches in his waist.

While Jason believes healthier eating is the foundation of his weight-loss success, he says he can't imagine achieving–or maintaining– his new lifestyle without regular exercise.

"I know that physical activity will need to continue to be a part of my life," says Jason. "Fortunately, it's something I enjoy and look forward to. I love the way I feel after I work out. The sense of pride and accomplishment is more satisfying than any meal I've ever eaten. I figure I'm going to have this body for the rest of my life. I want to give it the best care I possibly can."

Your Turn

Living With Gratitude

Today I live my life with an attitude of gratitude.

Today I am grateful for_____

_____

_____

_____

_____

_____

_____

_____

_____

_____

_____

DAY 26

"Wholeness lies beyond perfection. Perfection is only an idea. For most experts and many of the rest of us it has become a life goal. The pursuit of perfection may actually be dangerous to your health."

– Rachel Naomi Remen, M.D.

Find Something that Works

Dr. Remen is right. The pursuit of perfection *can* make the journey toward better health more difficult. Let me explain. Let's say that through much thought and trial and error, you create the perfect program of physical activity. Finally, you have the best possible plan. You begin the program and everything goes great. You follow it, you feel good, and you can measure positive results.

At some point, maybe as soon as a few days or as long as a few months, something will inevitably happen to disrupt your routine and derail your plans. No matter how much we deny or resist it, a simple fact of life is that life doesn't always go as planned. As one sage philosopher once observed, "Life is what happens while you're making other plans."

If you stop and think about it, you know exactly what we mean. Your child gets sick, your neighborhood is hit with the first hurricane in local history, your work hours are suddenly changed, or your bicycle gets stolen. You can no doubt add your own disruptions to this list.

When the inevitable happens and things change, you may have to "make do" with a less than perfect exercise program until you have a chance to create a new plan to incorporate the changes you're experiencing. This is very important. Instead of quitting, you keep going, even if what you're doing doesn't thrill you or suit you as well as you'd like. You accept life's imperfections and keep moving.

You may entertain yourself with dreams of perfection, but in the meantime, get out and take a 15 minute walk (instead of an hour), in the cold rain (instead of in the sunshine), at 5:30 in the morning (instead of in the evening as you'd prefer). Keep at it and do the best you can.

EAT BETTER: Whole Foods are Best

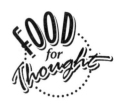

The scientific community recently has had another lesson in the value of eating real food, rather than just taking supplements. In 1977, when it became clear that beta-carotene helps decrease the risk of cancer and heart disease, people thought that taking beta-carotene supplements was the answer. It turned out, however, that supplements did not decrease the risk. In order to get the heart-saving benefits of beta-carotene, you needed to be eating yellow and green vegetables.

Why? Because real food contains hundreds of beneficial substances that aren't found in vitamin supplements. Our knowledge of what they are, what they do, and how they interact with each other is just beginning. We know that phytochemicals and antioxidants reduce the risk of cancer, and it looks like flavonoids prevent damage to blood vessels. It's no surprise that fresh fruits and vegetables (including soy) are great sources of these protective chemicals.

That isn't to say that vitamins are unnecessary. Unless you consistently eat a perfect, balanced diet of top quality foods, they are necessary. They just aren't *enough*. You still need to eat as many fruits, vegetables, and whole grains as you can.

"Negative thoughts are like pebbles. If you carry one or two around, you may not notice. But when you accumulate enough of them, they really weigh you down."

— Marshall B. Stamper, M.D.

MOVE MORE: Resistance Training

The more muscle you have, the more fat you'll burn. To make your body a fat-burning machine, add muscle-building exercises to your routine. Here are some simple resistance exercises that can be done with dumbbells, or even filled soup cans. The weight you use will depend on your level of fitness.

BUFF SHOULDERS

Here's a simple yet effective way to work your shoulder and trapezius muscles. Stand tall, with shoulders relaxed, and grasp a dumbbell or weight in your right hand. Slowly raise your arm away from your body and up toward the ceiling. You can bend your elbow slightly as you extend upward to shoulder height. For maximum benefit, concentrate on raising your arm slowly and smoothly. Hold for five to ten seconds, and slowly lower the weight. Repeat on the other side.

THE BACK OF YOUR UPPER ARMS

Hold a dumbbell in both hands behind your head with your elbows bent. With both upper arms staying steady at each side of your head, extend your arms upward so the weight is held over your head. Hold for five or ten seconds, and repeat.

ARM CURLS

Hold a dumbbell in front of you with both hands. Your elbows are slightly bent at your side, and your palms are facing out. Slowly bring the weight up to your chin. Hold for a few seconds, and slowly lower. Repeat. This exercise tones your biceps, the muscles in the front of your upper arm.

 STRESS LESS: A Letter of Appreciation

Have you ever written a letter of appreciation to a person or an organization to express thanks or support? Some of us are quick to voice complaints and criticism, but slow to express compliments or congratulations. There is no doubt the world is a better place when people take the time to let others know they see and appreciate the good work they're doing. When's the last time you said "Thank you", "I appreciate your efforts", or "Way to go!"? When you make an effort to help others feel good, you'll feel good, too!

Binge Eating Disorder

The American Psychiatric Association has proposed that binge-eating disorder be designated as a psychiatric disorder. What is binge eating disorder? Here are some common signs:

- *Eating rapidly.*

- *Eating several thousand calories in one sitting.*

- *At least two bingeing episodes a week for a period of at least six months.*

- *Bingeing alone and in secret.*

- *Feeling out of control during a binge.*

- *Feelings of self-hatred afterward.*

DAILY ACTION PLAN

Week _____   Day _____

Date _____   Weight _____

Breakfast Time:	Protein Grams	Fat Grams	Carbs Grams	Calories
Protein:				
Fruit:				
Grain:				
Beverage:				
Snack Time:				
Lunch Time:				
Protein:				
Vegetable:				
Lettuce:				
Grain:				
Fruit:				
Miscellaneous:				
Beverage:				
Snack Time:				
Dinner Time:				
Protein:				
Vegetable:				
Lettuce:				
Grain:				
Fruit:				
Miscellaneous:				
Beverage:				
Snack Time:				
TOTAL				

Today I was able to *Eat Better* by...

_____
_____
_____

Today I was able to *Move More* by...

_____
_____
_____

Today I was able to *Stress Less* by...

_____
_____
_____

Today I feel really great about...

_____
_____
_____

Tomorrow I will focus on...

_____
_____
_____

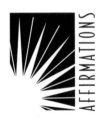

AFFIRMATIONS

"My body is strong and healthy."

• No purging, fasting, or exercise to compensate for the extra calories.

Binge-eating is an attempt to cope with emotions that are difficult or upsetting. Like anorexia and bulimia, the binger is involved in a secret, shaming obsession with food. But there are differences among these disorders. Binge eating is the more common affliction. While 2% to 5% of the population are binge eaters, 1% to 3% is bulimic, and less than 1% of the population is anorexic. Bingers are overweight or obese because they do nothing to compensate for the extra calories they consume, while bulimics are usually of normal weight because they fast or purge to compensate for extra calories. Anorexics are very thin because they are starving themselves. 90% to 95% of all anorexics and bulimics are female, while approximately two-thirds of binge eaters are female.

Tomorrow, we'll talk about what helps people who feel trapped in this nightmarish behavior.

Your Turn   Living With Gratitude

Today I live my life with an attitude of gratitude.

Today I am grateful for_____

_____

_____

_____

_____

_____

_____

_____

_____

_____

_____

DAY 27

"Why do we have to learn to recognize and assess our mood changes? Aren't most of us aware of our feelings at any given moment? Actually, it is the rare individual who characteristically knows exactly how she is feeling–and why–if you ask her without warning to describe her mood."
— *Lewis G. Maharam, M.D.*

A Well-Used Body

Children live in their bodies in a wonderfully natural and unselfconscious way. Few barriers block their free flow of feeling. As we get older, however, we have to work a little harder to inhabit our bodies with full awareness. It's so easy to become less aware and to start denying or distorting how well our bodies serve us.

This week's chapter is titled "The Beauty of a Well-Used Body," because it's important to emphasize that a body you live in is something beautiful. A body that moves, stretches, performs well and is pain-free is the best possible gift. To insist that your body conform to narrow media-driven standards in order to be appreciated is an insult to nature.

Your legs can be muscular or slender. Your skin can be freckled, tanned, or the texture of fine porcelain. You can have wrinkles or be wrinkle-free. Your legs may be long or short. What matters is that your body is well cared-for, and that it allows you to do what you want and need to do. The body of a newborn is a miracle, but so is the body of an older person.

It's important to develop an appreciation for real people and real bodies, and to embrace the breadth of bodily beauty we all represent. It's also essential that as a culture, we move away from the narrowly defined ideal of physical perfection that makes so many of us feel physically inadequate or even grotesque when we compare ourselves to it.

This change in perception begins inside each of us. As you follow your own program of better health, make it a point to notice and appreciate the beauty and miracle of your own body, and to do the same with others. Don't be bound by the artificial barriers of age and size. Think about what would happen if we all stopped insisting that beauty mimic the fleeting characteristics of youth. Aging would begin feeling more like an accomplishment to celebrate than a process to fear.

EAT BETTER: Help for Binge-Eaters

People who find themselves caught in out-of-control behaviors around food can be helped. Treatment involves a multi-tiered approach. Most important, perhaps, is learning how to identify your emotions and deal with them in an appropriate non-eating way. You must also learn how to eat appropriately in response to hunger signals instead of emotional triggers. And finally, it's helpful to have the opportunity to share your feelings with other people. Positive human relationships are an important part of recovery, since binge-eaters tend to be more depressed and isolated than non-bingers. In some cases antidepressant medications are prescribed and are helpful.

Here are three organizations that can give you more information:

- the American Anorexia/Bulimia Association at (212) 575-6200.

- the National Eating Disorders Organization at (918) 481-4044.

- Overeaters Anonymous at (505) 891-2664.

MOVE MORE: Yoga Breathing

Yoga was originally developed to make the body perfectly healthy so the practitioner could sit comfortably in meditation for long periods of time without bodily distractions. Both yoga and meditation are built on what is called "the complete breath." Deep, relaxing breathing nourishes your body and calms your spirit. Three complete breaths can be done before and after exercising as part of your warm-up and cool-down sessions.

These instructions for the complete breath are from the American Yoga Association:

- In a comfortable seated position, place your hands on the lower part of your rib cage, with your finger tips touching. Exhale fully, contracting your abdominal muscles.

DAILY ACTION PLAN

Week _____ Day _____

Date _____ Weight _____

Breakfast	Time:	Protein Grams	Fat Grams	Carbs Grams	Calories
Protein:					
Fruit:					
Grain:					
Beverage:					
Snack	Time:				
Lunch	Time:				
Protein:					
Vegetable:					
Lettuce:					
Grain:					
Fruit:					
Miscellaneous:					
Beverage:					
Snack	Time:				
Dinner	Time:				
Protein:					
Vegetable:					
Lettuce:					
Grain:					
Fruit:					
Miscellaneous:					
Beverage:					
Snack	Time:				
TOTAL					

Today I was able to *Eat Better* by...

_____
_____
_____
_____
_____

Today I was able to *Move More* by...

_____
_____
_____
_____

Today I was able to *Stress Less* by...

_____
_____
_____
_____

Today I feel really great about...

_____
_____
_____
_____

Tomorrow I will focus on...

_____
_____
_____
_____

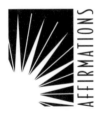

"I get all the rest I need so my mind and body are energized."

- Now relax your belly and inhale, pushing forward with your abdominal muscles and slightly arching your back.

- Continue to inhale, trying to expand your rib cage not just forward but also to the side. While still inhaling, straighten your shoulders and stretch your spine a little and feel the very top of your lungs. Your fingers should be moving apart. Then exhale.

Even beginners can feel the relaxing effects of this fundamental yoga technique.

STRESS LESS: Loving Through Listening

Listening with your undivided attention is one of the most healing acts you can perform for another person. Perhaps there is someone in your life who really listens to you, without interrupting or interjecting. If there is, then you know exactly what we mean.

Often, all we need in order to soothe our hurt feelings or calm ourselves is to have someone listen to what we have to say. We want someone to understand and share our feelings; we want to be heard and known by others. How strange, then, that we ourselves so often become careless with other people. Too often, we listen half-heartedly, or with an agenda of our own.

Make a promise to yourself today that you will bring your whole self to a conversation you have with someone who wants and needs your attention. While they're talking, don't compose a mental grocery list or prepare your response. Simply listen. Notice the healing effect your listening has on you as well as on your conversational partner.

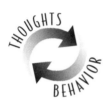

MENTAL FITNESS: Visualizing the Journey

Set aside ten or fifteen minutes today to visualize the journey you've already made toward better health. Reviewing how far you've come is a way to appreciate your resolve and your resilience as you go forward.

Let yourself be in a comfortable position. Close your eyes and take three complete breaths. Focus inward as you recall the moment or the occasion when you first decided to take control of your health. Let yourself see the scene and feel the feelings that energized you. Review the important steps you have taken since then. What are the pivotal moments in your efforts to eat sensibly and become more physically active? What scenes come to mind when you see yourself strengthening your relationship with yourself and with others? Take your time to relive the details of your progress.

After you've returned to your surroundings, think about the growth and the strength your story illustrates. Carry with you the lessons you think will be useful as you continue to become lean and fit and healthy.

Your Turn
Living With Gratitude
Today I live my life with an attitude of gratitude.

Today I am grateful for_____

_____

_____

_____

_____

_____

_____

_____

_____

_____

_____

DAY 28

"Whatever goes on in the mind has a direct effect on the body—and vice versa. An athlete's thoughts prompt certain emotions, and those emotions have physiological consequences."

– Tony Schwartz

Seeing with Different Eyes

Every journey, no matter where it takes you, is ultimately a journey inward. Every step you take shows you more about yourself and the way you live your life.

Many people have used physical activity as a means of self-discovery. People who climb mountains and explore remote and dangerous parts of the world learn a great deal about their personal strengths and values. But you don't have to be Edmond Hillary or Captain Cook to enjoy these experiences. Even the most humble exercise will give you insights you wouldn't have if you stay seated in your chair.

Most of these self-revelations will cluster around the realization that you can "do it"–whatever "it" is. You *can* stick to a routine. You *are* disciplined enough to exercise when you don't feel like it. Your body *does* have the capacity to become stronger. You *are* able to record your progress. You *can* enjoy setting new goals after you've achieved your earlier ones. You *do* love the self-confidence and high energy that fitness brings.

In addition to the undeniable physical benefits, being more active is a wonderful way to help strengthen your sense of self-mastery and self-awareness.

 ## EAT BETTER: Protein

You need protein every day. You can get it from meat, dairy products, or beans. In the past, you may have been tempted to get your protein from things like cheeseburgers, but now you can enjoy a soy burger, and benefit in many other ways as well. Here are some comparisons that may be useful:

- Two ounces of cheddar cheese gives you 14 grams of protein. But you also get 18 grams of fat, 12 of them saturated.

- Two ounces of broiled ground beef (about half of a regular sized hamburger) gives you 14 grams of protein. But you also get 10 grams of fat, 4 of them saturated.

- One whole soy burger patty provides 13 grams of protein, with only 1 gram of fat, and no saturated fat.

- One cup of cooked kidney beans provides 16 grams of protein, with only 1 gram of fat, and no saturated fat.

So look beyond grams of protein when making food choices. Just because a food offers lots of protein doesn't mean it's a healthy choice!

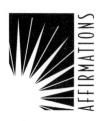

AFFIRMATIONS

"I enjoy physical activity and find many opportunities to exercise every day."

MOVE MORE: Exercise and Addictions

Exercise is vital for people recovering from addictions. Why? Alcohol and other drugs destroy the brain's ability to produce a balance of neurotransmitters that keep you feeling good and functioning well. Drinking and using drugs cause fluctuations in the brain's levels of norepinephrine, a neurotransmitter essential for emotional stability, and dopamine, which, when depleted, can cause paranoia, confusion, and memory loss.

When you stop dumping drugs into the system, your brain begins to restore its natural ability to regulate its delicate neurotransmitter system. And when you exercise, you help restore neurotransmitter levels to normal. The endorphins your body generates when you are physically active reward you with feelings of euphoria and well-being.

Exercise helps in other ways as well. It helps counteract the deadly effects of drug and alcohol addiction by improving your immune system, strengthening your muscles (including your heart muscle), improving coordination, lowering blood pressure, and decreasing cholesterol levels.

Clearly, moderate levels of regular exercise are important components in any recovery program.

STRESS LESS: Depression

Clinical depression appears to be the result of imbalances in brain chemistry, particularly low levels of norepinephrine and serotonin. Antidepressant drugs boost the levels of these two chemicals in the brain. People who are seriously depressed benefit from antidepressants and need them to return to full functioning.

But what if you are temporarily depressed or mildly depressed? What can you do for yourself? Current research supports these suggestions. Whether you'll want to do them instead of, or in addition to, antidepressant medication is a decision that needs to be made by you and your doctor.

- Get yourself outside. Sunlight entering your body through the retina of your eye will elevate your mood and increase your energy.

- Get moving. By now this is not a surprise to you. You know that exercise affects brain chemistry in such a way as to make you feel better.

- Meditate. Here, we include visualization/relaxation techniques, prayer, contemplation, and other forms of mental training. These are powerful ways of reducing stress and increasing your sense of well-being.

- Love. We're really talking about connecting in positive and meaningful ways with other people. Every time you have an interaction that lets you know that you are esteemed, understood, and valued, you are combating depression.

These are simple suggestions. They're yours to use. And they work. Think of other strategies you can use to make yourself feel better instead of blue.

How Do You Feel About Your Body?

In her book The Complete Idiot's Guide to Beating the Blues, *Dr. Ellen McGrath defines "Body Image Blues" as the negative feelings of shame, contempt, and disappointment in our bodies that most women and many men experience as they try to meet the unrealistic cultural standards of physical perfection, beauty, sex*

DAILY ACTION PLAN

Week _____   Day _____

Date _____   Weight _____

Breakfast Time:	Protein Grams	Fat Grams	Carbs Grams	Calories
Protein:				
Fruit:				
Grain:				
Beverage:				
Snack Time:				
Lunch Time:				
Protein:				
Vegetable:				
Lettuce:				
Grain:				
Fruit:				
Miscellaneous:				
Beverage:				
Snack Time:				
Dinner Time:				
Protein:				
Vegetable:				
Lettuce:				
Grain:				
Fruit:				
Miscellaneous:				
Beverage:				
Snack Time:				
TOTAL				

Today I was able to *Eat Better* by...

_____

_____

_____

_____

Today I was able to *Move More* by...

_____

_____

_____

Today I was able to *Stress Less* by...

_____

_____

_____

_____

Today I feel really great about...

_____

_____

_____

Tomorrow I will focus on...

_____

_____

_____

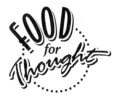

"We do not see

things as they are.

We see them

as we are."

— The Talmud

appeal, youth, and fashion. Do you have the Body Image Blues? Find out by taking Dr. McGrath's quiz. Answer "Yes" or "No" to the following questions.

1. Do you worry or obsess about the shape, condition, and/or size of your body every day?

2. Do you stand in front of a mirror and study your body for several minutes? Do you wish your body looked a lot different?

3. Do you feel fat no matter how much weight you lose or how much positive feedback you receive about your appearance?

4. Do you often feel intimidated by women or men you judge as thinner, stronger, better dressed, or more attractive?

5. Have you ever vomited or used laxatives to discharge food, or become so thin or heavy that your health has been affected (irregular or interrupted menstrual periods for women, impotence for men) because you were so unhappy with your body?

6. Do you feel frustrated that you "have nothing to wear" because you don't feel anything looks good on you, even though your closet is full of clothes? Do you feel clueless about fashion because you don't look like anyone on the cover of GQ magazine, even though your wife tells you which tie to wear?

7. Do you either dread the idea of shopping and trying on clothes or feel inadequate unless you're well dressed?

8. Have you ever seriously considered having a facelift, breast augmentation, penis enlargement, or any other elective cosmetic surgery because it would make you feel better about yourself?

9. Do you find that a new wrinkle, gray hair, or a few new pounds can wreck your day or morning?

10. Do you ever attempt to hide your body from your intimate partner or hide from yourself by avoiding looking in the mirror?

TOTAL NUMBER OF QUESTIONS ANSWERED "YES": _____

Do you have the Body Image Blues? Let's see how you scored:

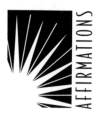

- 0-2: Congratulations! You've learned to love your appearance! If you scored within this range, you like the way you look and the way your body feels, even though you know it's far from perfect. You've somehow managed to duck the social pressures to look like an anorexic model or a body builder extraordinaire. The down side is that your friends probably wonder what's wrong with you, since you don't hate the way you look like all of them do.

- 3-5: Warning! You're prone to getting the Body Image Blues and may not realize when you're negative about your appearance. You get down on yourself because of the way you look more often than not.

- 6-7: Beware! You've probably got the Body Image Blues. You don't like how you look and go out of your way to do whatever you can to make up for what you think are your flaws and shortcomings. The body-perfect standard has really gotten to you, bashing you over the head with unrealistic expectations, and you must face up to your feelings or you'll feel worse and could develop a clinical depression or significant eating problems.

- 8-10: You're depressed. You haven't been able to escape the media and cultural image of how a woman or man should look and have taken to heart any bad things people have said to you about how you look. You may not even know how much you hate your body. But you do: BIG TIME! You could benefit greatly from professional help so your behavior can turn self-destruction into self-satisfaction. It may seem impossible, but you can learn to love your body regardless of age, stage, shape, or size.

If you answered "Yes" to two or more questions, you have some level of the body blues–but you don't have to have ANY of them. Just remember: You can reclaim your body from the crazy body-perfect standard of our culture.

WEEK 5

PROBLEM-SOLVING: The Ability to Figure It Out

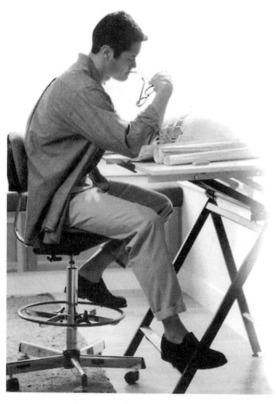

Your problems don't determine your success or failure. How you respond to them is much more significant. This week, you'll have the opportunity to develop winning attitudes and strategies that will help you become stronger because of your challenges.

DAY 29

"Acknowledge any stressful reality and see it as an opportunity to learn and grow. Quickly assess your alternatives and make the best decision based on the information you have. Then act. Even if you're feeling totally out of control, move with purpose and power as though you're completely in charge."

– Ellen McGrath, Ph.D.

Keeping At It

Wouldn't it be great if you could finish this maintenance business once and for all and never, ever have to think about it again?

Unfortunately, that's just not the way life works. In order to maintain, we must keep at it. As our lives change, we must find new ways to adapt. We change, therefore we must periodically reformulate our goals to keep them relevant and fresh.

How we view these challenges makes a tremendous difference. If, as Dr. McGrath suggests in the above quote, we learn to welcome stressful realities as opportunities to learn and grow, then we can learn to not be resentful and discouraged when they become apparent. We can learn to view obstacles as opportunities and problems as challenges. If it seems as though we have a lot to "learn", we do. We aren't born with the skills to immediately embrace and solve problems. Problems are, by definition, troublesome. But we can "learn" to make the best of what life gives us.

How do you want to deal with the problems that will inevitably come up? Do you want to develop an attitude of competence that says you can handle whatever challenges come your way, or will you allow yourself to feel beaten down and defeated when things don't go your way?

 ## EAT BETTER: Feeling Full

For a long time, people have known that a high fat diet is filling. Fat fills you up. But you may not know that a diet

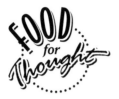

"Keep your face to
the sunshine and you
cannot see
the shadow."

— Helen Keller

high in water and high in fiber accomplishes the same thing in a much healthier way. That means that eating unprocessed or minimally processed fruits and vegetables and drinking lots of water or herb tea can be more satisfying than eating nonfat, processed snacks. It may take some getting used to. But trust me–it works!

So if you're worried about being hungry, think in terms of vegetable salads and fresh fruits–washed down with plenty of pure, unadulterated water. You'll feel comfortable longer, and you'll know that you are reaping all the other health benefits of eating well.

MOVE MORE: Maintaining Your Fitness Gains

Let's say you've been walking or working out in the gym for some months. You're now more fit than you've ever been. You feel good, and you look good.

But for any number of reasons, you find that your life changes and you can't devote as much time to your physical activity program as you have recently.

What does it take to maintain your aerobic gains? Fortunately, it only takes as little as three 20-minute sessions every week to maintain your fitness level.

It also doesn't take much to lose it. Your fitness level will begin to diminish after only two weeks of not exercising. And after five weeks of inactivity, you may very well find yourself at the same fitness level as before you began exercising. Obviously, it pays to keep going. But if you can't, don't stress out or be hard on yourself. As soon as you can, start over and enjoy the benefits of becoming fit all over again!

STRESS LESS: Giving It a Name

How are you feeling right now? Can you articulate your feelings and identify your emotions?

Most of us can say when we're mad, or sad, or happy, or afraid, but we have more trouble refining our descriptions beyond these broad categories.

Let's take "mad" as an example. People often tell themselves they're mad when what they really mean is that they're feeling disappointed, frustrated, surprised, insulted, fearful, anxious, or betrayed. While all are emotions, these feelings are very different from one another.

Why is this distinction so important? Because communicating clearly helps ensure that you're understood, and being understood is essential if

DAILY ACTION PLAN

Week _____   Day _____

Date _____   Weight _____

Breakfast Time:	Protein Grams	Fat Grams	Carbs Grams	Calories
Protein:				
Fruit:				
Grain:				
Beverage:				
Snack Time:				
Lunch Time:				
Protein:				
Vegetable:				
Lettuce:				
Grain:				
Fruit:				
Miscellaneous:				
Beverage:				
Snack Time:				
Dinner Time:				
Protein:				
Vegetable:				
Lettuce:				
Grain:				
Fruit:				
Miscellaneous:				
Beverage:				
Snack Time:				
TOTAL				

Today I was able to *Eat Better* by...

_____
_____
_____
_____
_____

Today I was able to *Move More* by...

_____
_____
_____
_____

Today I was able to *Stress Less* by...

_____
_____
_____
_____
_____

Today I feel really great about...

_____
_____
_____

Tomorrow I will focus on...

_____
_____
_____
_____

you and another person are determined to make positive changes in any relationship. Telling your partner you're angry, for example, may have undesirable consequences. Letting him or her know that you're feeling concerned or worried is likely to evoke an entirely different reaction.

The next time you're feeling any one of the big four (mad, sad, happy, afraid), see if you can be more specific. Pause for a moment to zero in on what you're really feeling. Learn to detect the subtleties, and more accurately name the gradations. It will then be easier to figure out appropriate responses to the feelings.

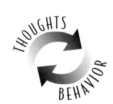

MENTAL FITNESS: What Makes People Stick to It?

Why do some people stick to exercise programs while others don't? This is the "$64,000 Question".

An interesting paper by E. A. Klonoff and others from the Behavioral Health Institute at California State University, San Bernardino, in March, 1994, addressed this question. The study enrolled twenty-three women in a free aerobics program in which they could attend as many exercise sessions as they chose. They recorded data about who attended the greatest number of sessions and who dropped out.

Those who attended the most sessions were overweight, shorter, had several physical complaints, and felt somewhat anxious. They concluded that psychological and physical discomfort predicted exercise adherence, and suggested that emphasizing the immediate symptom-relief benefits of exercise might help people in the general population begin–and stick with–an exercise program.

How can you use this information? Become sensitive to all the ways exercise gives you relief from physical and psychological symptoms. Record these observations on your Daily Action Plan, or in your journal. This will help you stay with it over the long haul!

DAY 30

"Pleasure is essential to most social activity. In the form of reward, it influences attachment and learning, particularly social learning, and willingness to participate in groups and obey rules."

– Peter D. Kramer

Reading the Signals

The inability to feel pleasure is a serious problem. Fortunately, it's an uncommon one. Most of us operate through a normal range of emotions, and come to trust that these emotions are giving us important clues about what we ought to do and what we ought to stop doing.

On the simplest level it seems obvious that we ought to do what feels good and stop doing what feels bad. Complications in this formula arise from the inborn complications of being human. For example, using drugs may feel good (in the present moment) but may end up making us feel very bad and being very bad for us. Jogging an extra mile may feel bad (in the present moment) but may end up making us feel good and be very good for us.

Nevertheless, even after acknowledging these complications, it still makes good sense to try to be in touch with all parts of our experience, particularly when we run into problems. An early warning system is a valuable weapon in the art of weight maintenance.

When something "doesn't feel right," take a moment to ask: Is there a problem? If there is, do I need to do something right now? Do I need to think about it first and then take action? You'll notice from these questions that you may not need to figure out a solution right on the spot.

First, just let yourself become aware of problems. Then practice a mental and emotional orientation toward the problem that is positive and confident (as we discussed yesterday). And *then* be smart about coming up with a solution.

EAT BETTER: The Paleolithic Diet

It's instructive to learn about how our human ancestors ate tens of thousands of years ago because it reveals important information about how our bodies have evolved and what kind of habits help our bodies work to maximum effect.

The human organism developed over millions of years to accommodate a low fat diet (approximately 20% of calories from fat) that was high in fruits, vegetables, fish, and meat. Scientists estimate that our ancestors ate about three times more fruits and vegetables (especially leafy, green vegetables) than we do. Since agriculture and the domestication of animals is very recent–only about 10,000 years ago–milk products and grains were unknown.

Only in the last 200 years have humans been able to eat as much fat, sugar, and energy-dense carbohydrates as they want. Since evolution proceeds in terms of hundreds of thousands of years, our biology has not caught up with our modern habits. It's no wonder that our high-calorie, high fat, and sugar-intense diets cause us so many health problems.

What fruits and vegetables are part of *your* menu plan today?

MOVE MORE: How Walking Combats the Common Cold

The good news about exercise just keeps on coming. Solid evidence now indicates that regular, moderate exercise, such as walking, bike riding, and aerobics helps you avoid the common cold. On those rare occasions when you *do* get sick, you will get over it faster if you are in the habit of walking or biking on a regular basis.

Moderate exercise boosts your immune system by increasing the number of white blood cells available to attack invading organisms. Although your white blood cell count returns to normal within hours of exercising, the temporary boost is enough to help cleanse your body of intruders.

If you're already suffering with a head cold, a walk can ease your symptoms. But if you have a fever, diarrhea, vomiting, coughing, or body aches, exercising can put too much stress on an already stressed system and make things worse. In that case, what you need is rest and plenty of fluids.

DAILY ACTION PLAN

Week _____ Day _____

Date _____ Weight _____

Breakfast Time:	Protein Grams	Fat Grams	Carbs Grams	Calories
Protein:				
Fruit:				
Grain:				
Beverage:				
Snack Time:				
Lunch Time:				
Protein:				
Vegetable:				
Lettuce:				
Grain:				
Fruit:				
Miscellaneous:				
Beverage:				
Snack Time:				
Dinner Time:				
Protein:				
Vegetable:				
Lettuce:				
Grain:				
Fruit:				
Miscellaneous:				
Beverage:				
Snack Time:				
TOTAL				

Today I was able to *Eat Better* by...

_____
_____
_____
_____

Today I was able to *Move More* by...

_____
_____
_____

Today I was able to *Stress Less* by...

_____
_____
_____
_____

Today I feel really great about...

_____
_____
_____
_____

Tomorrow I will focus on...

_____
_____
_____
_____

STRESS LESS: The Three-Minute Time Out

We all experience times when we're overwhelmed by anxious and stressful thoughts. We get caught in a raging current of worries that sometimes leaves us feeling as though we're about to drown in our own troubles.

You need to remember that there is always a way out. You can intentionally create a mental exit for yourself that will break the cycle of anxiety and distress. Here's how to do it.

- Recognize that you are caught in an anxiety avalanche and decide to take a time out.

- Close your eyes and shift your focus away from your upset emotions.

- Imagine your body bathed in a warm golden light that sustains you.

- Call to mind an image that calms you and gives you peace.

- Focus on this image and let your body experience its power.

- Listen to whatever message comes from within you and seems to answer the situation or person who is stressing you.

- Let yourself savor the words that come from your own inner wisdom and vow to carry them with you as you return to your surroundings.

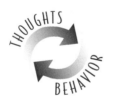

MENTAL FITNESS: A Meditation for Perspective

When the stresses and obligations of your life are too much, take ten or fifteen minutes out for this meditation.

Close your eyes and breathe three complete breaths. Imagine yourself floating on a soft, white cloud that cushions you and keeps you safe. You can float comfortably at just the right temperature, able to breathe freely and see as far as you want. At first you are hovering just above the earth at the level of a hot air balloon. Gradually, you rise higher and higher, and the earth recedes to a round ball. As you float further and further through space, you can see the entire solar system moving through the universe. Then you can envision your safe passage through the far reaches of the Milky Way and beyond. You experience the vastness of the universe and the miracle of the billions of stars that inhabit it. You realize that you are participating in the great stream of creation that is larger and more wondrous that you can ever imagine.

Carry these feelings with you as you return to your surroundings. Give yourself a few moments to think about how much you can know and yet how small you are in the total picture.

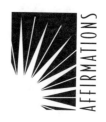

AFFIRMATIONS

"I take pleasure in doing what is good for me."

Your Turn. Living With Gratitude

Today I live my life with an attitude of gratitude.

Today I am grateful for_____

_____

_____

_____

_____

_____

_____

_____

_____

_____

_____

DAY 31

"Intelligent managing is based on the ability to take an objective look at a situation, to gather information, and then to react accordingly."

— *Mark H. Anshel*

An Objective Look

One way to take an objective look at what's happening in your life as it relates to food is to review your food diary section of your Daily Action Plans. If you don't like what you see, pinpoint the discrepancies between what you've *been* doing and what you *want* to be doing. Create a plan to close the gap and then implement your plan.

It sure sounds simple enough, doesn't it? In fact, you may be thinking that it's too simple. After all, in modern life where we have so many choices, our relationship with food can be as complex as any other aspect of our lives. But we also recognize the value of simplicity when it comes to problem-solving.

Recognize the problem. Generate solutions. Choose which solution is the best fit. Implement the solution. Whatever you do, don't forget to pat yourself on the back when it works!

EAT BETTER: Cutting Back After You've Overindulged

As you know, the art of maintenance is balance. This is especially true when it comes to food. There will be times when you consume more calories than your guidelines allow. You may want to indulge yourself at a special event or simply let yourself go for no particular reason.

You can relax and enjoy yourself better when you know that you will be able to tighten up and compensate the next day or the day after. If Saturday was a day of pancake breakfasts and barbecued ribs, for example, then Sunday can be a protein day. You can substitute a protein drink for one, two, or all of your three meals and know that you will be within your calorie budget for the week.

You can't live your life on a rigid schedule, but you can live within a margin of flexibility that allows you to make adjustments as you need to.

MOVE MORE: Increasing Your Activity After You've Overindulged

Part of your balancing act is learning to flex your activity level. In the same way that you can adjust your calorie level for any given day to be in balance for the week, you can walk extra steps, or put in extra minutes at the gym when you need to.

One of our patients loved having a fresh bagel every afternoon at the end of her work day. She had kept such good records that she knew a 45-minute walk every day made it possible for her to eat comfortably and have her bagel–and still maintain her weight. If she didn't walk, she didn't eat the bagel. It was that simple!

She had accumulated years of self-knowledge and knew what worked for her. You may not be so finely tuned. But even if you aren't yet, a good rule of thumb is to decrease your calories and increase your exercise after a day or two of extra eating. If you are weighing regularly and keeping good records, you will know how to adjust your eating and exercise to balance the unevenness of real life.

STRESS LESS: Loving Yourself Anyway

Darn it! You blew it! Either through oversight or choice, you didn't do the best thing, the thing you promised yourself you would do, no matter what.

Welcome to the real world. If you're honest and you're human, you're going to blow it sometimes. We all do. The idea that it's possible to walk a straight line from here to there is a fantasy. The question isn't whether or not you'll stray off the path, the question is: What will you do when you *do* stray?

You can certainly feel bad about it. That's okay as long as it doesn't last too long. If you find yourself feeling guilty, you may be overdoing it. If you find yourself paralyzed as a result, *then your reaction to the slip is worse than the slip itself.*

The next time you blow it, watch how you react. If you learn something from it and immediately start over again, then you are strengthening yourself over time. If you feel bad and then go crazy, you'll have to ask yourself whether you aren't being self-destructive.

So what do you think? Will you pay attention to how you respond the next time you blow it?

SUCCESS STORY: Ivy Williams

THEN&NOW

For four years, Ivy Williams dreaded the notion of going to the doctor for her annual check-up. After gaining a total of 80 pounds during two pregnancies, Ivy, who stands 5'2", was nearly 100 pounds overweight. She was well aware of the health risks associated with obesity, and was afraid any news her doctor might have for her wouldn't be good.

"I've seen what obesity can do to people in terms of heart disease and high blood pressure." says Ivy, 32. "I kept telling myself I should go, but I never got around to it. I allowed my fear over how my weight might be impacting my health to actually impact my health care."

When Ivy celebrated her thirtieth birthday, she decided it was time to take control of her weight, her body, and her health. "I knew that the longer I waited, the harder it would be to lose weight," she explains. "I also knew that the health risks associated with being overweight would be much greater as I got older."

When she began the Lean for Life program in April of 1997, Ivy weighed 229 pounds. In less than a year, she lost 95 pounds and has maintained at her goal weight ever since. These days, she is determined to do whatever she can to maintain her goal weight and enhance her health.

"After having avoided dealing with my health for so long, it feels terrific to be proactive," she says. "I do everything I can to stack the deck in my favor. I eat better than I ever have, I walk, run, bicycle, or use the stairmaster four times a week for at least 45 minutes, and I drink at least 80 ounces of water a day. I have a much better understanding of how my

DAILY ACTION PLAN

Week _____ Day _____

Date _____ Weight _____

Breakfast	Time:	Protein Grams	Fat Grams	Carbs Grams	Calories
Protein:					
Fruit:					
Grain:					
Beverage:					
Snack	Time:				
Lunch	Time:				
Protein:					
Vegetable:					
Lettuce:					
Grain:					
Fruit:					
Miscellaneous:					
Beverage:					
Snack	Time:				
Dinner	Time:				
Protein:					
Vegetable:					
Lettuce:					
Grain:					
Fruit:					
Miscellaneous:					
Beverage:					
Snack	Time:				
TOTAL					

Today I was able to *Eat Better* by...

_____

_____

_____

_____

Today I was able to *Move More* by...

_____

_____

_____

Today I was able to *Stress Less* by...

_____

_____

_____

_____

_____

Today I feel really great about...

_____

_____

_____

Tomorrow I will focus on...

_____

_____

_____

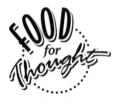

"Mistakes are a fact of life. It is the response to error that counts."

— Nikki Giovanni

body works and what it needs to operate most efficiently. I take care of myself in ways I never did before."

She says her newfound approach to eating and exercise has had a positive effect on her mental health, too.

"I have a lot more energy and a lot more self-confidence," Ivy says. "I feel a lot better about myself, and I feel like I'm setting a good example for my kids. When you succeed at a major goal like losing nearly 100 pounds, you gain a sense of inner strength that spills over into other areas of your life. It's very empowering."

It's that inner strength that makes it easy for Ivy to avoid the chronic temptation she faces nearly every day. Her 11-year-old son is an actor on a television series, and she spends most of her days on the set, where a buffet brimming with donuts, cookies, muffins, chips and other high-calorie, high fat foods is readily available.

"I've learned that the best way for me to eat well is to always be prepared," she says. "When I was on my weight loss program, I always prepared my food and took it with me. That way, I had choices. I still do that. Whenever I'm tempted to reach for food I know isn't good for me, I ask myself this question: 'Do you want to eat that stuff and be unhappy about the way you look and feel, or eat healthy and look and feel terrific?' When I put it in those terms, the answer is always simple."

DAY 32

"Remember, we are in charge of our own lives. If other people or circumstances are perceived to be in charge, then we are giving away what power we have. We can change. And we are well worth the effort and courage to change what we can."

David Miller and Kenneth Blum, Ph.D.

You Can Change

In fact, the truth is that you *will* change whether you want to or not. How you feel about this truth depends on the degree of choice you feel you have. When your long-time lover leaves, you may resist the change and try to hold on to him or her with all your might. But after awhile, when you realize that you are no longer such a dependent person, you may rejoice in this change toward independence.

Maintenance focuses primarily on positive changes that you *choose* to make. This kind of change requires effort on your part and persistence over long periods of time. Long-time maintainers often experience positive changes in eating and physical activity. After awhile, for example, they realize that they are no longer seeking emotional comfort from food and that they can act on their desires to take a bike ride or go on a long hike instead. They feel good about these changes and feel more empowered to make others.

There are aspects of your life you simply cannot change. You didn't choose your parents, for example. Your genetic inheritance may include a tendency toward obesity, and that may mean you have to work harder to maintain a healthy weight than your naturally skinny neighbor. You also can't change the fact you weren't born with the innate height to play professional basketball or that you're left-handed or have brown eyes.

Part of maintenance is knowing what you *can* change, what is *important* to change, *how* to change–and then letting the rest go. That's right–let it go. Do what you can do, learn how to enjoy what you have, and let the rest go.

EAT MORE: Intentional Eating

Every so often, you want to be able to eat whatever you want, whenever you want. But most of the time, you want to choose your food and the amount you eat with these three questions in mind:

1. How much energy have you expended during the day? If you've walked for an hour, you can eat more. If you've decided to take it easy, you can adjust accordingly.

2. How hungry are you? You can tune into your physical hunger signals and eat when your body needs fuel and not just when your emotional state compels to you get a food fix.

3. What is your body telling you would taste good right now? Consider the possibility that your body knows what it needs and learn to be responsive to that information.

By paying attention to these three factors, you can help restore your healthy relationship with food and counterbalance the food cravings that lead to both bingeing and starving.

MOVE MORE: Starting Over

You've developed a physical activity plan that really works for you. You look for opportunities to increase your activity, and engage in some intentional form of exercise five or six days a week. You're doing great!

And then, something unplanned and unexpected happens in your life and your exercise routine is suddenly interrupted. You pull a muscle while skiing; your great-aunt dies and you go out of town to attend the funeral; you buy a house and get tangled in the red tape of escrow.

When things finally settle down, it's tempting to start right in again on your exercise program where you left off. You remember the pleasures and benefits of exercise, and you're eager to experience them again. But if you don't allow yourself some time to ease back into where you were before you quit, you can easily injure yourself and really slow yourself down.

Whenever you're restarting an exercise program, be conservative. How conservative depends on your level of fitness, how long it's been since you exercised, and the details of your situation. Let's say you haven't exercised for two weeks and that when you stopped, you were exercising one hour a day.

DAILY ACTION PLAN

Week _____ Day _____

Date _____ Weight _____

Breakfast Time:	Protein Grams	Fat Grams	Carbs Grams	Calories
Protein:				
Fruit:				
Grain:				
Beverage:				
Snack Time:				
Lunch Time:				
Protein:				
Vegetable:				
Lettuce:				
Grain:				
Fruit:				
Miscellaneous:				
Beverage:				
Snack Time:				
Dinner Time:				
Protein:				
Vegetable:				
Lettuce:				
Grain:				
Fruit:				
Miscellaneous:				
Beverage:				
Snack Time:				
TOTAL				

Today I was able to *Eat Better* by...

_____
_____
_____
_____

Today I was able to *Move More* by...

_____
_____
_____
_____

Today I was able to *Stress Less* by...

_____
_____
_____
_____

Today I feel really great about...

_____
_____
_____

Tomorrow I will focus on...

_____
_____
_____
_____

How would you ease back into it? Start by exercising for 30 minutes today. If you feel fine, take another 30 minute walk tomorrow. If you still feel fine, increase your walking time for the next two days to 40 minutes. Then take a day off. The following two days, increase your time to 50 minutes. In just one week, you'll be back up to speed, walking a pain-free, injury-free hour a day.

If you think about it, taking one week to get back up to speed isn't much, especially when you consider the health risks and potential consequences of doing too much too soon.

STRESS LESS: We Are All Connected

Allow yourself to set aside ten minutes today for meditating on your loving relationships. When you are alone and free of distractions, close your eyes, let go of any bodily tension you may be feeling, and envision yourself as the hub, or the center, of a wheel. Spaced along the circumference of the wheel are several people with whom you feel especially close. You are connected to each of them by a line, or spoke, that goes from you in the center to each of them along the edge of the circle. As you draw an imaginary line from yourself to each person, take time to see each one of them in your mind's eye. Let yourself feel how much you love and appreciate each of these people, and the value you place on the invisible lines of connection that hold you together.

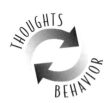

MENTAL FITNESS: Making Friends with Your Body

Many of us declare war on our bodies very early in life. We hate our thighs or our noses or our height or the color or texture of our hair or the way that one tooth angles to the left. We judge our bodies much more harshly than we'd judge nearly anything else.

A major step toward becoming a healthy person is undoing this damage and making peace with your body. After years of such harsh judgment, accepting your physical reality may not happen immediately, but it can be done. Generally, it is done in two parts: you stop the negative judgment, and you start verbalizing appreciation.

In order to stop body-bashing and break the cycle of negativity, you must catch yourself *before* you pass judgment so that the familiar litany of complaints doesn't get triggered. So many of our harsh comments are no more than knee-jerk reactions. It's as though we've *learned* to start moaning at the thought of buying a bathing suit or getting undressed in front of other people.

But if we learned it, we can *unlearn* it. Be aware of what situations trigger your negative thoughts and prepare for them ahead of time. Forewarned is forearmed. Commit to saying and thinking only positive things about your physical self and the way you look. Stop disparaging your body. You are in the process of making and maintaining healthy changes in your body. Focus on those improvements and rejoice in your progress. You'll be surprised at how the absence of negativity creates room for appreciation to begin to grow.

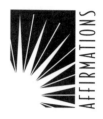

AFFIRMATIONS

"I am enjoying my new sense of well-being."

Your Turn.

Living With Gratitude

Today I live my life with an attitude of gratitude.

Today I am grateful for_____

_____

_____

_____

_____

_____

_____

_____

_____

_____

_____

_____

DAY 33

*"No defeat is made up entirely of defeat–since
the world it opens is always a place unsuspected."*
– William Carlos Williams

The Value of Failure

Failure is never fun, but it doesn't have to be a wasted experience. In fact, many of history's extraordinary people have written that they learned more from their mistakes than they ever did from their successes.

While success merely confirms what you already thought you knew, failure provides you with new information. It's important to keep asking yourself what you're learning when things don't go as you had hoped, planned, or expected. Your answers will help shape your thinking and allow you to come up with new solutions you wouldn't have thought of before.

Let's test this theory. Look back in your Daily Action Plans and identify one eating "failure" and one activity "failure" from the past month. Now think carefully about what each failure taught you. Be as specific as you can. Can you identify how this new insight or piece of information shaped your thinking from that point forward?

Let's say your food diary shows you went from 11:30 in the morning until 5:30 one night without eating. The "failure" was that you allowed yourself to become famished and gobbled down 2,000 calories worth of fast food as you drove home from work. What you learned was that you need to have at least one snack (and possibly two) in order to feel under control later in the evening. If you pay attention, those 2,000 calories you squandered actually taught you a lot.

 EAT BETTER: Using Structure to Support Yourself in Shaky Times

Many people manage to stay on an eating program just fine until something stressful happens in their lives.

Suddenly, their commitment and best intentions are eclipsed by familiar and often unproductive eating habits. What if, when life got stressful, we learned to rely on the healthy routines we know work for us? What if instead of breaking down, we recommitted to the sensible plans and programs we constructed in easier times.

Is your relationship with your partner on thin ice? Take extra good care of yourself by nourishing your body well. Is your boss being especially demanding and unappreciative? Maintain your balance by paying special attention to your eating and exercise program. Does your future feel out of control? Take charge of one of the few things that is totally under your control and eat as though your good health depended on it–which it does!

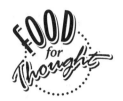

"The game of life is a game of boomerangs. Our thoughts, deeds, and words return to us sooner or later, with astounding accuracy."

– Florence Scovel Shinn

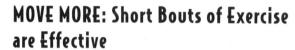

MOVE MORE: Short Bouts of Exercise are Effective

In 1995, a study found that obese women who did several short bouts of exercise during the day (about 10 minutes for each session) were more likely to stick with it than those who exercised in one long session. In addition, short bouts of exercise also appeared to enhance weight loss, and produced the same level of cardiovascular fitness as one long session.

This is important information. It means that 10 minutes of walking, biking, or marching in place several times a day really makes a difference. You don't have to walk 30 minutes at a time to gain value from exercise. Stop whatever you're doing right now and move your body for ten minutes. When you're finished, notice how you feel.

STRESS LESS: The Two-Minute Retreat

This suggestion is from Jennifer Louden's *The Woman's Retreat Book: A Guide to Restoring, Rediscovering, and Reawakening Your True Self–In a Moment, an Hour, a Day, or a Weekend.*

• Take five deep, cleansing breaths. Drop your jaw. Breathe into your belly. Run your fingers through your hair. Move your shoulders toward your ears, tense, and release. Repeat three times.

• Imagine yourself wrapped in a cone of protective white light.

- Imagine the light entering your body through the crown of your head. Or, if you can, stretch your arms over your head, and imagine that you are bringing this brilliant, healing light into your body through your outstretched hands.

- Allow light to penetrate to wherever you feel tired, anxious, sad, or worried.

- Smile and say silently to yourself, "This is the present moment. There is goodness in this present moment. I trust myself to find it."

- Feel grateful for the light that has warmed you, and imagine it condensing into the palm of your hand so that your palm glows with warmth and power. Place your hand over your heart or clasp your hands together.

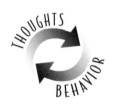

MENTAL FITNESS: Three Internal Challenges that are Related to Lapses

According to James Prochaska in his book, *Changing for Good*, there are three mind games that people play when they are subconsciously courting relapse. Awareness of them and vigilance against them will help you continue to maintain your weight within an acceptable, healthy range.

1. Overconfidence. If you think you can relapse into the behaviors that caused your problem in the first place and not be sucked back in, you're probably setting yourself up for a fall.

2. Placing yourself in the path of daily temptation. You can see how the first and second are related. Overconfidence can lead to temptation. People who fill their homes with high fat food and "experiment" with taking a week off from exercise will discover that sooner or later, temptation wins and they lose.

3. Self-blame. It can be a good thing to realize when you have messed up and to use that realization to get yourself back on track. But if you consistently feel bad and guilty about yourself, you are sapping valuable energy away from the effort you need in order to move yourself forward.

DAILY ACTION PLAN

Week _____ Day _____

Date _____ Weight _____

Breakfast	Time:	Protein Grams	Fat Grams	Carbs Grams	Calories
Protein:					
Fruit:					
Grain:					
Beverage:					
Snack	Time:				
Lunch	Time:				
Protein:					
Vegetable:					
Lettuce:					
Grain:					
Fruit:					
Miscellaneous:					
Beverage:					
Snack	Time:				
Dinner	Time:				
Protein:					
Vegetable:					
Lettuce:					
Grain:					
Fruit:					
Miscellaneous:					
Beverage:					
Snack	Time:				
TOTAL					

Today I was able to *Eat Better* by...

_____

_____

_____

_____

Today I was able to *Move More* by...

_____

_____

_____

Today I was able to *Stress Less* by...

_____

_____

_____

_____

_____

Today I feel really great about...

_____

_____

_____

_____

Tomorrow I will focus on...

_____

_____

_____

_____

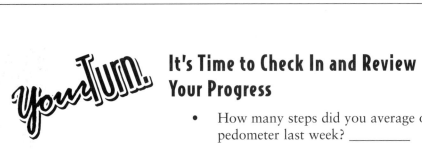

It's Time to Check In and Review Your Progress

- How many steps did you average on your pedometer last week? _____

- Is your weight within three pounds of your weight on Day One? If not, what will you do for yourself today?

  _____

- Are you filling out your Daily Action Plan every day? _____

DAY 34

"You, too, will come to understand how your good food intentions can have unexpected outcomes and how your own relationship with food can negatively affect your daughter's."
— Debra Waterhouse, M.P.H., R.D.

Sabotage

It's hard to understand why someone who loves you would try to sabotage your efforts to maintain your new health habits. Surely your wife or your mother want what's best for you. Yet the fact is that sometimes the people we're closest to have the most difficult time adjusting to the positive changes we make in our lives. We change, and that sometimes requires them to change–whether they want to or not.

Our experience has shown that the best way to prepare friends and family to support you is, in fact, to prepare them. Tell them what you are doing. And tell them what you want from them. (That also includes telling them what you *don't* want from them.) In a perfect world, the people who love you would know what you want and need without your having to say one word, but that rarely seems to be the case.

Here's an example of how you can effectively communicate what you are doing and the support you would like the other person to provide:

- "I want to make some changes in the way I eat. I'm making an effort to eat less for dinner and to skip dessert until I achieve my goal weight." (This is a clear statement of your intentions.)

- "You can support me by understanding that when I don't eat a high fat dish you've prepared, it isn't because I don't like it or don't love you." (This is a clear statement of what you would like from the other person.)

Make a point to include lots of reassurance and appreciation in your conversation.

Is there someone close to you who seems to be sabotaging your efforts? Using the above example as a guide, what would you like to say to them? Once you've given it some thought, say it! It's the surest way to turn a saboteur into a supporter.

EAT BETTER: Saying "No, Thank You"

Sometimes it seems so hard to say "No, thank you" that we almost think of it as a major achievement, something only certain people are capable of. We imagine that it takes extraordinary finesse and skill, not to mention lots of practice. Actually, it doesn't have to be that difficult at all.

Here are some simple ways to turn down that piece of homemade chocolate pie or that second gin and tonic:

- "No, thank you. I've had all I want."

- "Thank you for asking, but I don't care for any."

- "That looks so delicious, but thanks anyway."

- "I'm very tempted. That looks so good. But no, thank you."

There are endless variations, all of which require a gracious and appreciative but direct demeanor. The real question here is whether you're going to please yourself or the person offering the food you don't want. Is it more important to say yes to your host or to stay committed to your own program? If you're appreciative and smile when you say "No, thanks", you'll feel better and your host will feel fine, too.

MOVE MORE: Self-Motivation

You know what it's like to have trouble getting motivated. All of us reach those times when we just don't want to do it anymore. We feel drugged into inaction by our own apathy or even antipathy.

Each of us has a private code of motivators that is as personal and unique as a fingerprint. These are the ideas, feelings, and images that get our blood going again. When we don't care anymore, these are the things that pique our interest.

Do you know what motivates you to be physically active when your interest is lagging? The best motivators are positive. Although fear of failure can be a powerful motivator, it's better to be moving *toward* something than away from something.

Here are some possible motivators. Take a moment to read through the list and mark the ones that work for you. Add your own to this list. The next time you feel lazy and unmotivated, they just might help you get up and moving.

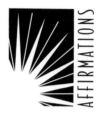

AFFIRMATIONS

"I like seeing myself as an effective problem solver."

Positive Motivators

- _____ I have more energy when I'm active.

- _____ I am less stressed when I'm active.

- _____ I am more patient when I'm less stressed.

- _____ My body looks better.

- _____ My body *is going to* look better.

- _____ I enjoy feeling disciplined.

- _____ I know I am doing good things for my general health.

- _____ I am setting a good example for other family members.

- _____ I enjoy knowing that I am caring for myself in an important way.

- _____ Other people's good examples motivate me.

- _____ Photos of what I want to look like motivate me.

Negative Motivators

- _____ I don't want to feel the way I once did.

- _____ I don't want to look the way I once did.

- _____ I don't want to feel out of control.

- _____ I don't want people to be disappointed in me.

- _____ I don't want to feel less confident about myself.

- _____ I'm afraid of the negative health consequences.

You can be motivated by anything. Find out what works for you–whether it's a photograph taped to your bathroom mirror, a daily affirmation, a review of the positive health benefits, talking with other people–and *do those things that keep you focused on your goal.*

 ## STRESS LESS: Positive Self-Talk, Part 1

How would your life be different if you were perfectly content and at peace? Imagine appreciating all your working parts and enjoying the way you look and feel. When you look around, you feel that your body is just as beautiful as anyone else's. And when you open the pages of magazines or watch movies, you don't feel intimidated by images of beautiful women or handsome male models.

Pause for a moment and let yourself imagine such a world. Then ask yourself how you would think, feel, and act differently. How would you live if you had no body hatred? Then take a vow that you are living in such a world for just one day. Let yourself feel contentment as you get dressed in the morning. Allow yourself to be confident that every part of you is acceptable, if not beautiful.

When you do talk to yourself about your appearance, speak loving words. Float your body in a cloud of appreciation. "I look just the way I should look. My body works wonderfully well, and I am grateful. I have a right to wear these clothes and to be expressive in my choices. I have a right to be free of the self-imposed burden of disapproval that I've been carrying around."

Find your own words of freedom and appreciation and then flood yourself with them. Start with just one day, and then, if you like how you feel, say it all over again on the second day, and the third, and the fourth. . .

SUCCESS STORY: John Morgan

When John Morgan lost 75 pounds on the Lean for Life program three years ago, he knew that maintaining his weight loss would require the same level of commitment as losing it. But what he didn't anticipate

THEN&NOW

was the subtle sabotage from friends and family that he says made maintaining his weight loss a major challenge.

"I've been amazed at how eager people seem to be to fatten me up," says John, a general contractor and father of two. "Ever since I lost the weight, many of the people in my life constantly encourage me to eat. They say things like 'C'mon, you've earned it' or 'One piece of chocolate cake won't kill you'."

John is convinced that the commitment and discipline he developed while on his weight loss program made some of his friends, business colleagues, and family members feel self-conscious and uncomfortable.

"They say misery loves company, and I really think that's true," says John. "When you're around someone who's really making progress, it makes you that much more aware that you're standing still. I think people find it threatening when someone is succeeding in an area in which they feel inadequate or undisciplined."

Even John's wife and kids encouraged him to eat more.

"My wife accepts me whether I'm fat or thin, but I honestly think she prefers it when I'm heavier," says John. "And my kids definitely do. One of them actually said to me, 'Dad, we really miss your Santa Claus tummy. It was a great pillow when we watched TV.'"

Last Christmas, the saboteurs won—at least temporarily. John finally surrendered to temptation.

"I bought into the notion that I could 'treat' myself during the holidays," he recalls. "The irony is that after I lost the weight, I never really missed junk food. But once I started binging on sweets again, I went ballistic."

DAILY ACTION PLAN

Week _____   Day _____

Date _____   Weight _____

Breakfast	Time:	Protein Grams	Fat Grams	Carbs Grams	Calories
Protein:					
Fruit:					
Grain:					
Beverage:					
Snack	Time:				
Lunch	Time:				
Protein:					
Vegetable:					
Lettuce:					
Grain:					
Fruit:					
Miscellaneous:					
Beverage:					
Snack	Time:				
Dinner	Time:				
Protein:					
Vegetable:					
Lettuce:					
Grain:					
Fruit:					
Miscellaneous:					
Beverage:					
Snack	Time:				
TOTAL					

Today I was able to *Eat Better* by...

_____

_____

_____

_____

_____

Today I was able to *Move More* by...

_____

_____

_____

_____

_____

Today I was able to *Stress Less* by...

_____

_____

_____

_____

Today I feel really great about...

_____

_____

_____

_____

Tomorrow I will focus on...

_____

_____

_____

_____

In eight months, John regained 26 pounds.

"I was disgusted that I allowed myself to fall back into the same old patterns," he says. "I stopped exercising, stopped maintaining a food diary, and basically stopped taking care of myself. The good news is that I finally realized where I was headed and was able to say, 'I'm not going to let that happen' before I put all 75 pounds back on."

John recently began the Lean for Life program again to lose the 26 pounds he regained.

"It's been a humbling experience, but it's also been a valuable life lesson," he says. "Because I lost the weight so easily, I think I took my weight loss success for granted. But knowing how much better I look and feel when I'm not heavy is a real motivation to get back down to a weight where I feel healthy and attractive. This time, I'm going to stay there."

YourTurn. Living With Gratitude

Today I live my life with an attitude of gratitude.

Today I am grateful for_____

_____

_____

_____

_____

_____

_____

_____

_____

_____

_____

_____

DAY 35

"The healthier people, when they find their present ways of life dull, frustrating, or tedious, pay attention to their 'all is not well' signals and change what they are doing, including their ways of behaving with others."

– *Sidney M. Jourard*

Appreciate the Negative

Trying to avoid unpleasant feelings and circumstances isn't an especially successful strategy for living. In fact, many people come to realize that an inability to deal with negative emotions is part of why they put on excess pounds in the first place.

You don't have to promote conflict or even welcome it. But when it does arise, you can accept it and see what can be learned from it. A good way to start is to try hearing the critical comments of people around you in a neutral way that provides you with new information. Try listening instead of denying and defending. After you've really heard the message, you have a choice whether to accept or reject all or part of what you've heard. But before you make that decision, you first have to hear what's being said.

What you'll discover is that accepting negative information as you go along will help you make changes that will prevent catastrophes later. When people feel they can give you critical feedback in bits and pieces, they don't bottle-up their resentments until they explode into more serious eruptions. And when you give yourself the same permission to give others feedback in bits and pieces, you provide yourself with an escape valve that makes it easier for you to stay balanced and focused on your own goals.

 EAT BETTER: Gains Through Grains

Grains are an important part of a healthy diet. Consider the following:

- All grains are carbohydrates, but not all carbohydrates are grains.

- Simple carbohydrates are sugars. Complex carbohydrates, including grains, are found in bread, cereals, pasta, and rice.

- Complex carbohydrates take longer to digest and provide more continuous energy than sugar.

- A gram of carbohydrate contains 4 calories, less than half the calories found in a gram of fat.

- Examples of grain-based foods are rice, oatmeal, grits, barley, pretzels, bread sticks, rolls, granola, bulgar, pizza, polenta, bagels, muffins.

- Some examples of one serving of grains: one small tortilla, one slice of bread, half a bagel, one small waffle, half a cup of cooked pasta, 4 saltine crackers, 3 fig bars, one small muffin, or one 4-inch pancake.

What grains have you included on *your* menu plan for today?

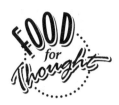

"Think only the best, work for only the best, and expect only the best."

— Christian D. Larsen

MOVE MORE: Cross-Training

Variety, it's said, is the spice of life. That's especially true when it comes to exercise. Varying your exercise program so you don't do the same day after day is a smart way to prevent injuries and boredom. While many people like to vary their activities so they're swimming one day, biking another day, and walking the next, it is possible to cross-train within the same family of exercise.

For example, here are three different activities that can be done in an aerobics class to music with a group of other people:

- Step-aerobics: Stepping up and down on an elevated platform in time to music.

- Weights: Lifting wrist or hand weights in time to music as part of floor exercises.

- Toning: Doing floor exercises such as abdominal curls, leg lifts, or toe touches in rhythm to the music.

Variety strengthens all parts of your body, and ensures that you're practicing a full range of motion in all your muscle groups. There are also psychological benefits of doing different things on different days. If you have three ways of getting your exercise, you'll have three different activities to be interested in and to master.

STRESS LESS: Positive Self-Talk, Part 2

If your body supports your weight and allows you to move pain-free, then it is working well for you. If your body is free from disease and you feel well, then it is working well for you. If your body helps you experience a full range of emotions, including joy, then it is working well for you.

A body that works well is worth celebrating. Many people aren't so lucky. Through illness, accidents, and age, they've become prisoners in their own bodies, unable to move freely. As part of your celebration, vow to spend a couple of minutes every day appreciating your body for the things it does so well. You can write a couple of sentences in your journal or say to yourself the things you are grateful for.

Be thankful that you can reach up to the top shelf for a bottle of soy sauce. You can bend down and scoop a child into your arms. You can walk for an hour. You can feel the rush of sexual excitement. You can sleep when you're tired. Focus on what your body does, not just on how you think it looks.

When All's Not Well

Having one of those days? One of those weeks? When all's not well, remember that getting active makes a big difference in how you feel. These "action strategies" from Dr. Ellen McGrath's book The Complete Idiot's Guide to Beating the Blues, *will help.*

- *When you're blue, identify what's triggered your bad mood if you can do so right away, otherwise put that off until you feel better.*

- *The Action = Energy = Power formula says that every action you take creates energy, and as your energy builds so does your power and potential to meet your goals.*

- *Identify a goal a day to keep you focused and help you feel productive.*

DAILY ACTION PLAN

Week _____   Day _____

Date _____   Weight _____

Breakfast	Time:	Protein Grams	Fat Grams	Carbs Grams	Calories
Protein:					
Fruit:					
Grain:					
Beverage:					
Snack	Time:				
Lunch	Time:				
Protein:					
Vegetable:					
Lettuce:					
Grain:					
Fruit:					
Miscellaneous:					
Beverage:					
Snack	Time:				
Dinner	Time:				
Protein:					
Vegetable:					
Lettuce:					
Grain:					
Fruit:					
Miscellaneous:					
Beverage:					
Snack	Time:				
TOTAL					

Today I was able to *Eat Better* by...

_____

_____

_____

Today I was able to *Move More* by...

_____

_____

_____

Today I was able to *Stress Less* by...

_____

_____

_____

_____

Today I feel really great about...

_____

_____

_____

_____

Tomorrow I will focus on...

_____

_____

_____

_____

- *To perk you up when you're feeling low, take a ten-minute walk instead of grabbing a candy bar or drinking a double espresso.*

- *Helping others makes you feel capable, kind, and giving–all feelings that will enhance your self-esteem.*

- *Deep breathing, meditation, and positive visualization techniques transport you to a calm, relaxed, and blissful state.*

- *Keeping a journal is an effective form of self-therapy and helps you sort out your thoughts.*

WEEK 6

MENTAL STRENGTH: The Key to Change

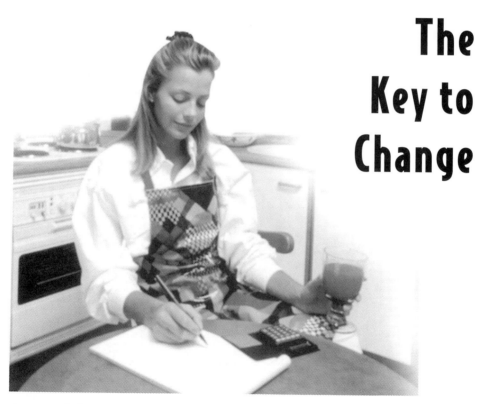

Successful people develop mental strength. As any Olympic athlete will tell you, while part of every performance is physical, a greater part is mental. This week, you will learn how you can become more focused, more disciplined, and more resilient.

DAY 36

"Morrie had begun to cough while eating, and chewing was a chore. His legs were dead; he would never walk again. Yet he refused to be depressed. He jotted down his thoughts on yellow pads, envelopes, folders, scrap paper. He wrote bite-sized philosophies about living with death's shadow. 'Accept what you are able to do and what you are not able to do;' 'Accept the past as past, without denying it or discarding it;' 'Learn to forgive yourself and to forgive others;' 'Don't assume that it's too late to get involved.'"

– Mitch Albom

What Do You See for Yourself?

People who function exceptionally well in life are mentally strong. They've developed an innate ability to focus and can often work for long hours without tiring. They've developed these abilities over years of intentional *practice*.

There's another aspect of their lives that isn't always apparent: They nearly always have a strong vision of what they want for themselves in the future. They "see" themselves functioning in certain ways, and they imagine themselves achieving certain goals.

The athlete sees herself breaking the record. The businessman sees himself building his profits. The artist sees herself achieving the technique that pushes her art to a new level.

It's useful for all of us to ask ourselves what we see in our own futures. We have it within us to adopt an attitude that assumes that whatever we see is achievable and that, even if we don't know how we are going to solve the inevitable problems, we *will* be able to get there from here.

Where do you see yourself one year from now? Take fifteen minutes and imagine where you'll be–and what it will take to get you there.

EAT BETTER: Accepting, Not Fighting

People who have successfully lost weight and kept it off are rarely at war with themselves over food anymore. They've come to terms with whatever changes they have to make in their foods habits. They live comfortably and steadily with moderation. Some of them have eliminated red meat or butter or ice cream altogether, while others continue to allow themselves on occasional treat.

Imagine what it's like to be off the food roller-coaster, to know what you *can* eat, what you *want* to eat, and to find pleasure in that. You too can do it, and you can start today. Like all habits, eating in moderation and with a conscious awareness of food choices requires focus, determination, and commitment.

MOVE MORE: Move and Live

According to the Iowa Women's Health Study, postmenopausal women who engage in moderate physical activity more than four times a week may reduce their risk of death by more than one-third compared to women who aren't active. "Moderate" activity included bowling, golfing, gardening, and walking. Even exercising as little as once a week lowered the risk of death by 24%. Vigorous activity, such as swimming, aerobics, jogging, or racquet sports, afforded the most protection. But not everybody wants to run four miles everyday. And guess what? You don't have to. What would you *like* to do today? Go do it!

STRESS LESS: The Power of Words

If you could read a transcript of the things you say to yourself in the privacy of your own mind, would you be pleased with what it said? If you saw in black and white the words you use in the stream of your own consciousness, would you be pleased by the caring and encouraging way you move yourself through your own experience, or would you would be dismayed at the harsh, even abusive, way you approach your life?

Learning how to "read" your own internal messages is a useful skill to develop. The next time you forget to do something, or the next time you say something inappropriate, listen to the words you use when you talk to yourself about it. Are you saying, "Darn. Everyone makes

DAILY ACTION PLAN

Week _____   Day _____

Date _____   Weight _____

Breakfast	Time:	Protein Grams	Fat Grams	Carbs Grams	Calories
Protein:					
Fruit:					
Grain:					
Beverage:					
Snack	Time:				
Lunch	Time:				
Protein:					
Vegetable:					
Lettuce:					
Grain:					
Fruit:					
Miscellaneous:					
Beverage:					
Snack	Time:				
Dinner	Time:				
Protein:					
Vegetable:					
Lettuce:					
Grain:					
Fruit:					
Miscellaneous:					
Beverage:					
Snack	Time:				
TOTAL					

Today I was able to *Eat Better* by...

_____

_____

_____

_____

Today I was able to *Move More* by...

_____

_____

_____

_____

Today I was able to *Stress Less* by...

_____

_____

_____

_____

Today I feel really great about...

_____

_____

_____

Tomorrow I will focus on...

_____

_____

_____

_____

mistakes. I usually do a better job. I'll do better next time."? Or are you saying, "You Idiot! You always do that. You're hopeless!" ?

If you think you're a hopeless idiot and you keep reinforcing that idea with your negative self talk, it's likely that you'll continue to act in the same manner and continue getting the same result. It's a vicious cycle. But you can change your self talk. Mental strength is like physical strength. It takes practice–lots of it!

SUCCESS STORY: Tammy Randall

One of Tammy Randall's prized possessions hangs on the refrigerator of her Thousand Oaks, California home. It's a school essay that her daughter, Kaitlyn, wrote two years ago when she was just six. It reads: "My mother is loving. She is the best. She is fun. She is skinny and she eats well."

When she looks at that piece of paper, Tammy, 38, can't help but grin. For most of her life, she wasn't "skinny" and didn't "eat well" at all. The mother of six, Tammy's weight hovered at 175 pounds for more years than she cares to count. After her last two pregnancies, she found it increasingly difficult to lose the "baby weight". At 5'8" she weighed 210 pounds and had grown increasingly unhappy and frustrated with her body.

"I was well aware that my weight had gotten out of control, but when you have six kids, you're so busy running from school to soccer practice to piano lessons that it's easy to put off taking care of yourself," she explains. "I knew that one day I'd do something about it. I just wasn't sure when that day would come."

That day came one October afternoon when Tammy received a phone call informing her that her oldest son, Larry, had broken his neck in a wrestling accident while away at college in Boston. She hopped a plane and spent the next month away from the daily frenzy of activity that had become her life. While providing moral support to her son at the hospital, she was forced to face a health issue of her own.

"The first time I climbed the stairs in the hospital, I thought I was going to die," she recalls. "I was totally out of breath and my heart was beating so hard that you could see my chest moving. One of the nurses actually asked me if I was feeling all right. I live in a one-story house and work at a one-story office, so it had been a very long time since I'd climbed a flight of stairs. I knew I was out of shape, but that was a real eye opener."

During the four weeks she spent at the rehab facility, Tammy had plenty of time to reflect on life and how she was living hers.

"I remember looking around and thinking to myself that I was the luckiest person in that room," she says. "My son was showing real signs of progress, and except for the extra sixty pounds I was carrying, I was healthy. So many of the people I saw were facing health challenges they weren't going to conquer. My weight–my health–was something I could do something about."

Tammy's son amazed his doctors by making a full recovery, and Tammy amazed herself when, six months later, she lost 59 pounds and achieved her goal weight of 150 in just twelve weeks. She has stayed within two pounds of her goal for more than two years.

"They say that life is what happens while you're making other plans," Tammy reflects. "One of the lessons I learned is that we don't have nearly as much control in our lives as we often think we do, but there are some things we *can* control. One of them is what we eat and how well we take care of ourselves. That's something I'll never take for granted again."

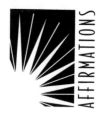

AFFIRMATIONS

"Challenges make me stronger."

DAY 37

"If the world were perfect, it wouldn't be."
— *Yogi Berra*

The Perils of Perfection

One characteristic of mental strength is the capacity to roll with the punches. Instead of needing the world to be a certain way, highly successful people learn to expect the unexpected and not be thrown off by surprises. One place where it's easy to see the role of serendipitous discovery is in the area of science. Most of our important discoveries–penicillin, for example–were accidents.

This theme often plays out in film and novels–you know, the ones where the boy would never have met the girl if he hadn't missed the bus and come in out of the rain for a cup of coffee and sat next to her at the diner. Some people call it happenstance. Others call it dumb luck.

Whatever you call it, the bottom line is that the world wouldn't be perfect if it *were* perfect because nothing new, nothing magically unexpected and surprising, would happen. The wild and wonderful creative element that makes life interesting would be missing. The universe isn't a machine; it's a living organism like us.

Can you think of something unexpected–either "good" or "bad"–that happened to you in the last week or two? Was there anything you would have, or could have, done differently?

 EAT BETTER: Another Food Myth

"A candy bar or a piece of chocolate is an energy booster." There was a time when swimmers and other competitive athletes believed this old wives tale and were encouraged by coaches to eat sweets before a major race or competition.

We now know that eating a candy bar causes a slow rise in blood sugar (glucose), not a quick increase as once believed. In response to the rise in blood sugar, your body produces insulin. The insulin acts to lower glucose levels either by directing it to the muscles to be burned as fuel, or to fat cells to be stored if your muscles aren't being used enough to require extra fuel.

The best way to ensure a constant flow of energy throughout the day is to eat regular, balanced meals and snacks, get enough sleep, drink enough water, get enough exercise, and to do some relaxation and visualization exercises.

Remember: the state of your body is a reflection of everything you do *for* it, *with* it, and *to* it.

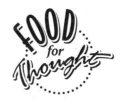

"Our greatest fear isn't that we are inadequate. Our deepest fear is that we are powerful beyond measure. It is our light, not our darkness, that most frightens us."

— Marianne Williamson

MOVE MORE: The Aging Process Can be Slowed—or Even Reversed

The USDA Human Nutrition Research Center on Aging at Tufts University has unearthed surprising evidence that many aspects of the body's decline are due to inactivity, poor nutrition, and illness. They are not the inevitable and inescapable consequences of getting older.

Their research has shown that with only 50 minutes a day of aerobic exercise and strength training, middle-aged and older adults can:

- Regain lost muscle and increase their strength by as much as 200%.

- Reenergize the body and lose body fat.

- Increase aerobic capacity up to 20%.

- Reduce the chances of developing conditions such as heart disease, Type II diabetes, and osteoporosis.

Increasing your physical activity and making dietary changes can go a long way toward preserving health into old age. These lifestyle habits are within your control. You're never too old to exercise and to start eating better. Every positive change you make will help you traverse the latter part of your life with strength, energy, good health, and a lean body.

DAILY ACTION PLAN

Week _____   Day _____

Date _____   Weight _____

Breakfast Time:		Protein Grams	Fat Grams	Carbs Grams	Calories
Protein:					
Fruit:					
Grain:					
Beverage:					
Snack Time:					
Lunch Time:					
Protein:					
Vegetable:					
Lettuce:					
Grain:					
Fruit:					
Miscellaneous:					
Beverage:					
Snack Time:					
Dinner Time:					
Protein:					
Vegetable:					
Lettuce:					
Grain:					
Fruit:					
Miscellaneous:					
Beverage:					
Snack Time:					
TOTAL					

Today I was able to *Eat Better* by...

_____

_____

_____

_____

_____

Today I was able to *Move More* by...

_____

_____

_____

_____

Today I was able to *Stress Less* by...

_____

_____

_____

_____

Today I feel really great about...

_____

_____

_____

_____

Tomorrow I will focus on...

_____

_____

_____

_____

STRESS LESS: I See You and I Appreciate You

You've undoubtedly heard the expression that you can attract more flies with honey than with vinegar. It's true. You'll attract more with a loving outlook than a with a disparaging one, more with an open heart than with a judgmental one. You'll find more love, more creativity, and more humor in your life when you share these qualities with others.

Today, make it a point to tell your child, your partner, or another significant person in your life one specific thing that you love and appreciate about them. You can give your five-year-old a hug, look into his face, and say, "I really like it when you tell me what happened at school today." Or you can squeeze your wife's hand and say, "I really love it when you . . ."

Expressions of appreciation and love are like a cool drink on a sweltering day. It's hard to get too much.

Your Turn   Living With Gratitude

Today I live my life with an attitude of gratitude.

Today I am grateful for_____

_____

_____

_____

_____

_____

_____

_____

_____

_____

_____

_____

DAY 38

"Without a good dose of curiosity, wonder, and interest in what things are like and how they work, it is difficult to recognize an interesting problem."
— *Mihaly Csikszentmihalyi*

Life Force

Curiosity is another characteristic of mental strength. We all know people who seem to have been born with an extra measure of life force. They're highly energetic, interested in the world around them, and indomitable in their high spirits and determination. And we all know people who are fragile, disinterested, and spiritless.

The study of human biology is showing that some of these characteristics are built into our genes. You may have heard people talk about what's being called the "happiness gene." People who possess it seem to maintain a high level of happiness and contentment, no matter what happens to them. In fact, their happiness in general seems to function somewhat independently of actual events.

Biology aside, however, there are certain predictors of high energy. As you review them, think about how many apply to you. People with high vitality are generally:

- physically healthy.

- exercising regularly.

- loved and are loving.

- believing in what they are doing.

- spiritually alive.

- rested.

How many of these predictors of high energy are within your control? You can't do much about your biology and whether or not you were blessed with the "happiness gene". But you can cultivate these other components of vitality. That's what this program is all about—offering strategies you can work on for enhancing your energy levels, enhancing your health, and enhancing your life.

EAT BETTER: All Beef is Not Created Equal

If you've decided to eat vegetarian, that's fine. But you don't have to give up beef entirely if you don't want to. Nowadays, ranchers are breeding leaner cattle. In fact, the leanest cuts of eye round, top round, top sirloin, top loin, tenderloin, and others with the words "loin" and "round" in the name, can have as little saturated fat as chicken and turkey. (Hamburger does not qualify.) And there are some important vitamins and minerals in beef, including five B vitamins, zinc, iron, and B-12 that you can't get from plants.

MOVE MORE: Before and After

According to a recent poll of fitness trainers, the most common error people make when they work out in the gym is not stretching after a workout. Stretching after exercise is vital because it keeps your muscles flexible and can help prevent soreness, stiffness, and injury.

Warming up *before* you exercise is also important. Warming up means gradually increasing your breathing, your body temperature, and the blood flow through your muscles. Motion that is easy and controlled prepares your muscles to stretch even more and to work harder and longer. Warming up also aids in flexibility and helps prevent injuries.

Just a few moments of special attention to your muscles before and after you exercise can make a real difference.

STRESS LESS: The "We-ness" of Me

Personal development always involves some sort of evolution from an I-centered view of the universe to a more we-centered view. One indication of where you are along the path toward self-discovery is to listen to yourself talk.

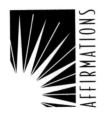

"I appreciate my body and feel good about the changes I see."

How often do you say "I" when you could (or should) be saying "we"? How willing are you to include others in the stories you tell about your life? When there is praise, do you share it? When you've borrowed a phrase or a concept, do you give credit? Sharing the blame, of course, is another matter. Often, the noblest thing to do is share the credit and take the blame. This doesn't weaken you; it makes you stronger.

The next time you begin to notice that your conversation is all about you, ask yourself whether it isn't more honest and more gracious to make it more about "us." Then notice if you feel different when you talk "we" instead of "me".

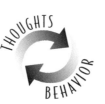

MENTAL FITNESS: Sex and the Immune System

The more we know about the way our bodies and minds work, the more in awe we are about how beautifully everything fits together. By staying close to the path that nature intended, we stay healthy and hearty.

There's a reason sex feels so fabulous. First, it has to feel good in order to insure the continuation of the species. If it didn't feel good, we wouldn't want to do it. But beyond that, it feels good because it *is* good for us. The sexual response involves all of our body systems, including our immune system. Hormones interact with neurotransmitters to give us a sense of well-being. Our beating hearts keep our circulation healthy. The exercise keeps our bodies strong and flexible. Heavy breathing sends oxygen through our bodies and helps release carbon dioxide. We look better, we feel better, and there is a spring in our step.

In addition, there are several recent studies which seem to demonstrate that sex strengthens immune function. It has been found that women with breast cancer who describe their sex lives as excellent have a higher number of T-cells (white blood cells that fight invaders) than women who have no sex life or consider their sex lives to be unsatisfactory.

DAILY ACTION PLAN

Week _____   Day _____

Date _____   Weight _____

Breakfast Time:		Protein Grams	Fat Grams	Carbs Grams	Calories
Protein:					
Fruit:					
Grain:					
Beverage:					
Snack Time:					
Lunch Time:					
Protein:					
Vegetable:					
Lettuce:					
Grain:					
Fruit:					
Miscellaneous:					
Beverage:					
Snack Time:					
Dinner Time:					
Protein:					
Vegetable:					
Lettuce:					
Grain:					
Fruit:					
Miscellaneous:					
Beverage:					
Snack Time:					
TOTAL					

Today I was able to *Eat Better* by...

_____

_____

_____

_____

Today I was able to *Move More* by...

_____

_____

_____

Today I was able to *Stress Less* by...

_____

_____

_____

_____

Today I feel really great about...

_____

_____

_____

_____

Tomorrow I will focus on...

_____

_____

_____

_____

DAY 39

"After the first moments of fear have passed, the long haul of survival begins, perhaps to the accompaniment of hunger, thirst, pain, and adverse weather. A crucial survival tool will be a reasoning mind, one that is able to view the ordeal not as an overwhelming set of threats but as a puzzle to be solved."

— *Time Life Books*

How You Think of It

A reasoning mind is able to think clearly under a variety of conditions. While there is no way to separate thoughts from feelings, it is possible not to let your emotions cloud your thinking. In high-stress situations, people who function best are those who think clearly no matter what.

Reason is also a useful tool for ordinary living, not just extraordinary situations. Being able to think up practical strategies for solving everyday problems helps you stay on your maintenance program. Here are some brief examples of rational attitudes that help people succeed:

- "I'm not sure yet how I'm going to solve this problem, but I know I'll figure it out."

- "I wish I hadn't done that, but I'm not going to let it ruin the rest of my week. I'll do what I can to fix it and move on."

- "My first reaction is that this is going to upset me. But I know that in a while, I'll calm down and sort out what to do."

- "I can't do this all by myself. I need to ask for help."

- "I'm really sorry that this is happening to you, but I know that it's not my problem."

EAT BETTER: Cutting the Fat

Cutting down on fat and using your calories for nutritious food is an important element in maintaining your weight. Most maintainers find that they can't continue using high fat flavorings such as butter on their bread, sour cream on their baked potatoes, and blue cheese dressing on their salads. They limit or even eliminate their use of such flavorings.

In fact, a study published in the May 1992 *Journal of the American Dietetic Association* found that women who were trying to restrict their fat intake to no more than 20% said that avoiding fat as a flavoring was the single most important step they took in maintaining a low fat regimen.

There are a variety of low fat options available now. You can experiment with low fat mayonnaise, nonfat sour cream, fat free salad dressings, and diet margarine. Admittedly, the change in taste takes a little getting used to. Eating your bagel plain instead of with cream cheese is an adjustment. But you can do it. How much is it worth to you to be lean for life?

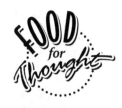

"We could never learn to be brave and patient if there were only joy in the world."

— Helen Keller

MOVE MORE: Exercise and Weight Maintenance

In 1997, the *American Journal of Clinical Nutrition* published a study that examined the link between physical activity and weight maintenance, and how much physical activity was required to optimize maintenance.

Researchers found that it took an average of 80 minutes a day of moderate activity or 35 minutes a day of vigorous activity, added to a sedentary lifestyle, to maintain weight. In order to lose weight, 45 minutes of exercise, such as brisk walking, seven days a week, was necessary. Women who were physically active at the time they reached their target weight gained fewer pounds during the next year than those who were less active.

STRESS LESS: Love Yourself into Something Better

Psychologists Murray Millar and Karen Millar have shown that people are more likely to change their behavior when they are moving toward positive goals than when

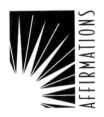

"I can grow in mental strength as I grow in physical strength."

they're frightened and attempting to move away from the negative. People who read statements saying that at some point they would eventually develop a serious disease were less able to think about taking positive steps than those who read statements about the importance of staying healthy to pursue important goals.

How can you use this information? First, you can apply the suggestions in this book to help you encourage rather than discourage yourself. Second, you can keep alive the vision of yourself as lean and healthy.

You can make your maintenance program a positive and exciting adventure of self-discovery. Plot your successes, and then enjoy them!

MENTAL FITNESS: Mindfulness

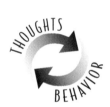

The practice of mindfulness helps you focus on whatever you're doing at the moment so you are concentrating fully on the activity you're engaged in. Instead of being only partially present, you're fully focused whether you're shopping for groceries, comforting a crying child, or performing demanding tasks at work.

Jon Kabat-Zinn, Director of the Stress Reduction Clinic at the University of Massachusetts Medical Center, has developed an exercise in mindfulness called "The Raisin Exercise." Eating mindfully involves holding your food, feeling it, noticing its texture, becoming aware of how it grew and where it came from. These instructions are adapted from Dr. Kabat-Zinn:

- Pick up a single raisin and look at it very carefully. Notice the color, the peaks and valleys of its texture, the degree of shininess, and its shape and size. Smell it and notice the aroma. Lick it, and place it in your mouth. Hold it there without chewing while the flavor pervades your mouth. Savor the taste for at least one minute. Slowly begin to chew the raisin, perhaps 30 or 40 times, while the flavor blossoms. At last you can swallow, being aware of the remnants on your teeth, and the flavor that lingers on your tongue.

- Take your time with this exercise. The goal is to fully see, taste, and feel what you are doing. Being mindful of eating a raisin is good practice for being attentive to all the other moments of your day.

DAILY ACTION PLAN

Week _____ Day _____

Date _____ Weight _____

Breakfast	Time:	Protein Grams	Fat Grams	Carbs Grams	Calories
Protein:					
Fruit:					
Grain:					
Beverage:					
Snack	Time:				
Lunch	Time:				
Protein:					
Vegetable:					
Lettuce:					
Grain:					
Fruit:					
Miscellaneous:					
Beverage:					
Snack	Time:				
Dinner	Time:				
Protein:					
Vegetable:					
Lettuce:					
Grain:					
Fruit:					
Miscellaneous:					
Beverage:					
Snack	Time:				
TOTAL					

Today I was able to *Eat Better* by...

_____
_____
_____
_____

Today I was able to *Move More* by...

_____
_____
_____
_____

Today I was able to *Stress Less* by...

_____
_____
_____
_____

Today I feel really great about...

_____
_____
_____
_____

Tomorrow I will focus on...

_____
_____
_____
_____

DAY 40

"Your brain holds a rich vault of knowledge and wisdom that, at this moment, may be partially inaccessible to you because your memory and cognitive powers may be starved, battered, or underdeveloped. But that wealth of understanding is definitely there, very much alive, physically encoded, virtually immortal, waiting for you to reach it."
— Dharma Singh Khalsa, M.D.

Getting Stronger

The way you get stronger is to use your mental muscles. Like the body, the mind also responds positively to the stress of exercise.

If you lived in a hermetically sealed environment where nothing was ever asked of you, and if you had all your needs taken care of, you wouldn't be able to cope if someone suddenly dumped you onto the street. You learn to function well in the course of meeting challenges.

Admittedly, it is important that you consider the challenges to be worthwhile and that they be manageable. When stress upon stress is piled on until you feel overwhelmed, that's as likely to have a negative effect as a positive effect on your overall mental health.

But that aside, the problems you're asked to solve every day give you a chance to build new neuronal pathways in your brain that open up capacities you didn't have before. You can't play the violin without ever having practiced. And you don't become an expert problem-solver without having problems to solve.

EAT BETTER: Reading the Record

Have you reviewed your Daily Action Plan lately? If not, this is a good day to review your eating records.

Here are some questions you can ask yourself:

- Are you eating enough so that you're not hungry?

- Are you staying within your guidelines? (Do you need to modify your guidelines?)

- Are there times when you eat more than you needed or wanted? Do you know why? Did you write about it in your Daily Action Plan?

- Are you eating in a balanced and nutritious way?

- Are there changes you need to make?

Your Daily Action Plan is an invaluable record of this very important part of maintenance. It can encourage you, and also help you make corrections. Every so often, you need to pause long enough to stop and notice the message.

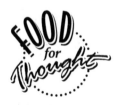

"The battle to keep up appearances unnecessarily, the mask—whatever name you give creeping perfectionism —robs us of our energies."

— Robin Worthington

MOVE MORE: Exercise and Breast Cancer

In 1997, a Norwegian study found that physical activity can reduce the risk of breast cancer. During a 14-year study of more than 25,000 women, ages 20 to 54, those who engaged in at least four hours of moderate exercise a week were 37% less likely to develop breast cancer than women who were sedentary.

STRESS LESS: Your Journal

Writing in your journal has cumulative benefits. The more you write, the more you'll deepen your awareness of what is happening in your life. If it's been awhile since you allowed yourself this reflective pleasure, here are some ideas:

- Write about how you felt after finishing a vigorous workout.

- Write about how you felt when you last dealt successfully with a food craving.

- Write about the last time you felt like crying.

- Write about one thing you want to accomplish during the next week.

SUCCESS STORY: Richard Evanns

THEN & NOW

If it weren't for a cement wall on a Southern California college campus, 19-year-old Richard Evanns might still weigh 310 pounds.

"I used to jump over this four foot high wall as a shortcut to my girlfriend's apartment," he explains. "It saved me a lot of time and a long walk."

But one day, Richard recalls, it seemed as though the wall had magically grown.

"We'd been away on summer break for a few months, and the first time I tried to hop over the wall in September, I really had a tough time," he says. "I told myself I must just be tired. But when it didn't get easier, I realized that the wall hadn't changed, but the body I was trying to put over it obviously had. It was a real wake-up call."

At the time, Richard didn't have a clue how much he weighed. He had weighed around 260 throughout high school, but didn't own a scale and hadn't weighed himself for two years. He guessed that he'd gained about 30 pounds, and was stunned when he hopped on the scale at his doctor's office and saw the number: 314 pounds.

Richard made a decision then and there to lose weight. And he did. He lost 101 pounds in 10 months and has maintained his loss for nine months.

While Richard says he never considered himself to be unhappy when he was heavy, he's the first to admit his life is healthier and happier today than ever before.

"I guess you could say that I didn't know what I was missing," he says. "I've heard all kinds of stories about how people felt so ugly and humiliated when they were fat. That wasn't my experience. I never felt like a victim, though now that I've lost weight, I notice a major difference in how I feel. I have a lot more energy and I'm more willing to do and try new things now. It's also a lot easier to buy clothes and feel like I look good."

The changes in Richard's lifestyle have been remarkable. These days, he works out at the gym and surfs three to four days a week.

"I hadn't been to the beach since junior high because I was self-conscious about taking my shirt off," he says. "I'm a lot more comfortable and confident about my body now."

DAILY ACTION PLAN

Week _____   Day _____

Date _____   Weight _____

Breakfast Time:	Protein Grams	Fat Grams	Carbs Grams	Calories
Protein:				
Fruit:				
Grain:				
Beverage:				
Snack Time:				
Lunch Time:				
Protein:				
Vegetable:				
Lettuce:				
Grain:				
Fruit:				
Miscellaneous:				
Beverage:				
Snack Time:				
Dinner Time:				
Protein:				
Vegetable:				
Lettuce:				
Grain:				
Fruit:				
Miscellaneous:				
Beverage:				
Snack Time:				
TOTAL				

Today I was able to *Eat Better* by...

_____

_____

_____

_____

Today I was able to *Move More* by...

_____

_____

_____

Today I was able to *Stress Less* by...

_____

_____

_____

Today I feel really great about...

_____

_____

_____

Tomorrow I will focus on...

_____

_____

_____

What people seem to notice even more than the change in his body, Richard observes, is the change in his attitude.

"People who have known me for a long time tell me that I'm more fun and outgoing, that I look and act like a different person," he says. "I like hearing that because it reminds me how much I've changed and how much progress I've made in a fairly short period of time. It feels terrific to have faced such a big challenge and to have succeeded this early in my life."

Your Turn. **Living With Gratitude**

Today I live my life with an attitude of gratitude.

Today I am grateful for_____

_____

_____

_____

_____

_____

_____

_____

_____

_____

_____

"Anything that promotes a sense of isolation leads to chronic stress and, often, to illnesses like heart disease. Conversely, anything that leads to real intimacy and feelings of connection can be healing in the real sense of the word: to bring together, to make whole."

– Dean Ornish, M.D.

Love

Dean Ornish, M.D. is a passionate and powerful advocate for the central role that love and intimacy play in healing. This is an idea most of us can support from our own personal experience, but Dr. Ornish has done a great service by supporting the notion with convincing research evidence.

Part of being mentally strong is loving–opening yourself to other people instead of closing yourself off–and being able to extend past your comfortable boundaries and risk new feelings and new choices.

This takes strength. Letting other people get close means that you learn how to meet someone else's needs when you'd rather not. And if you're lucky, it means that you stick around long enough to learn what it's like to be there over the long haul, even when the long haul is sometimes tiring or even boring.

Loving well makes you stronger, and we now know that it also helps you heal.

EAT BETTER: Food Boredom

Feeling bored with food is a privilege of the privileged. Not everyone has the luxury. Nevertheless, there are times in our privileged culture when the thought of eating the same old breakfast once again is just more than you can handle.

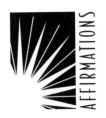

"I have confidence I will succeed."

Admittedly, some people have the same thing for breakfast or lunch every day for years and never protest, while others of us aren't happy unless each day represents a whole new adventure.

Because maintenance requires discipline and limits, it makes sense to set up a routine and follow it, at least for awhile. But when you feel yourself growing bored, do what you can to stir things up a bit. Here are a few ideas for breakfast to get your own gastronomic juices flowing:

- Substitute cottage cheese for yogurt.

- Make your usual fruit and yogurt into a smoothie by adding a little skim milk and blending in a blender.

- Try your poached egg with a little salsa.

- Get your vegetables by drinking a tall glass of salt-free or Light and Tangy V-8 juice.

- Have lunch for breakfast if you want to.

With a little imagination, you can break out of boring food patterns and keep things interesting.

MOVE MORE: Activity Boredom

Some people seem to have a far greater threshold for monotony than others. When it comes to exercise, they're so relieved to find something that works for them that they're willing to stick with it no matter how monotonous it becomes. But if you find yourself growing bored and restless and are looking to add some variety into your exercise, here are some ideas:

- Buy or rent a book-on-tape to listen to while you walk or use the exercise machines.

- Walk a different route.

- Exercise with a partner–or go solo for a change.

- Substitute another activity for your usual choice.

- Take your walk mindfully instead of in your usual distracted state.

DAILY ACTION PLAN

Week _____ Day _____

Date _____ Weight _____

Breakfast	Time:	Protein Grams	Fat Grams	Carbs Grams	Calories
Protein:					
Fruit:					
Grain:					
Beverage:					
Snack	Time:				
Lunch	Time:				
Protein:					
Vegetable:					
Lettuce:					
Grain:					
Fruit:					
Miscellaneous:					
Beverage:					
Snack	Time:				
Dinner	Time:				
Protein:					
Vegetable:					
Lettuce:					
Grain:					
Fruit:					
Miscellaneous:					
Beverage:					
Snack	Time:				
TOTAL					

Today I was able to *Eat Better* by...

_____

_____

_____

_____

Today I was able to *Move More* by...

_____

_____

_____

_____

Today I was able to *Stress Less* by...

_____

_____

_____

_____

_____

Today I feel really great about...

_____

_____

_____

Tomorrow I will focus on...

_____

_____

_____

_____

_____

- Break up your exercise into three 15-minute segments instead of doing it all at once.

- Join a fitness club and sign up for a class you haven't tried before.

- Do your weight lifting routine in a different order.

STRESS LESS: Don't Forget to Breathe

Full belly breathing is the fastest way to let go of tension. In the few seconds it takes to breathe in deeply five times, you can break the cycle of stress and muscle tension that tends to build up during the day without your realizing it.

If you haven't been practicing breathing every day, take the time to do it now. Close your eyes, let go of muscle tension, and breathe in for five deep breaths.

How do you feel now? From now on, remember that you have a fast, easy, effective tool for re-energizing yourself whenever you are feeling tired and tense.

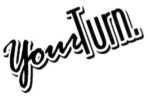

Maintaining Your Commitment

It makes sense to do what you can to maintain your commitment to living lean for life, rather than waiting until you're on a downward slide and then trying resurrect a plan later.

Make a point of setting aside fifteen minutes a week to review your commitment to your eating and exercise program. There are a number of ways you can do this. Write down the problems you encountered before you made positive lifestyle changes. Review the list. Remembering the misery of being fat and sedentary will help you keep up your new habits.

You can also write down the benefits and payoffs of your accomplishments. Describe in detail what it's now like to go clothes shopping, or how you feel on the tennis court. Immersing yourself in the joy of being fit and lean will help you keep up your new habits.

DAY 42

"What you are feeling is completely natural–it is the primal grasping of grief."

– Stephen Levine

Letting Go

Most of us think of getting stronger as building up, getting more, and being more, but it can also mean having less and letting go of attitudes, behaviors, and people who are negative and counterproductive to our growth and happiness.

As you think about your own path through maintenance, can you think of what you've had to give up or chosen to give up? Are there behaviors and activities you've had to leave behind as you continued to grow and develop? If these losses are clear to you, have you taken the time to mark their passing? Even the loss of behavior that didn't serve you well still needs to be acknowledged.

Take a moment now to reflect on what you've left behind. These are examples of what we are talking about:

- I no longer mindlessly eat in front of the TV.

- I no longer sleep in until 9:00 in the morning on weekends.

- I no longer party every weekend.

- I no longer order double-cheese pizza on Saturday night.

- I no longer make chocolate chip cookies for the kids and eat half the batter before it even gets into the oven.

Being aware of what you've chosen to let go and give up is the first step toward being grateful for the new things you've chosen to include in your life.

EAT BETTER: Food Isn't Everything

One of the things that happens when you regain control over food is that you begin to get pleasure from a lot of other aspects of your life. You broaden your base of happiness. You're not seeking happiness, enlightenment, and relief all in one place. Your senses come alive. Think about the pleasures of:

- A steaming cup of tea and one cookie.

- Shoes that are shined.

- An organized closet.

- A Beethoven sonata.

- Books in order on a shelf.

- The clouds in the sky.

- A pebble, any pebble.

Eating is one strand that is woven into a tapestry of pleasures that thread themselves all through your days and nights.

MOVE MORE: Moving On

Just for fun, decide to pursue one new form of activity this week. I'm not necessarily talking about taking kayaking or belly dancing lessons, although learning something new is a great idea if you have the time.

I'm suggesting something as simple as walking around the block on your lunch hour. Or jogging every second block during your walk. Or dancing to music in the afternoon for a few minutes. Or borrowing your daughter's jump rope and jumping for a bit. Or trying some of the stretches suggested in this book.

When you do something new, it makes you feel great. And it reminds you that there are many different opportunities for moving. You don't have to think along the same old paths. Try taking the road less travelled. You just may be amazed at the view.

DAILY ACTION PLAN

Week _____   Day _____

Date _____   Weight _____

Breakfast Time:		Protein Grams	Fat Grams	Carbs Grams	Calories
Protein:					
Fruit:					
Grain:					
Beverage:					
Snack Time:					
Lunch Time:					
Protein:					
Vegetable:					
Lettuce:					
Grain:					
Fruit:					
Miscellaneous:					
Beverage:					
Snack Time:					
Dinner Time:					
Protein:					
Vegetable:					
Lettuce:					
Grain:					
Fruit:					
Miscellaneous:					
Beverage:					
Snack Time:					
TOTAL					

Today I was able to *Eat Better* by...

_____
_____
_____
_____
_____

Today I was able to *Move More* by...

_____
_____
_____
_____
_____

Today I was able to *Stress Less* by...

_____
_____
_____
_____
_____

Today I feel really great about...

_____
_____
_____

Tomorrow I will focus on...

_____
_____
_____
_____

STRESS LESS: You Are Moving Forward

What do you consider your biggest achievement since you began your maintenance program? Maybe it's sticking to a regular exercise program or keeping daily records or making meditation a part of your life. On the other hand, you may feel really good about the way you are eating.

Because weight maintenance is a comprehensive activity, there are many different opportunities for doing things well and feeling good.

Take time today to think about the positive steps you are taking in your life. One large accomplishment may come to mind first, but then allow yourself the pleasure of reviewing all the little ways you are caring for your body, mind, and soul. There are so many. It will serve you well to be aware of all of them.

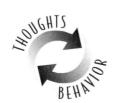

MENTAL FITNESS: Mental Imagery Can Distract You From Pain

One of the difficulties of chronic pain is that the pain can take on a life of its own. It's easy to become isolated in your own misery. Fortunately, researchers and clinicians have found that people who become involved in mental imagery can effectively distract themselves from mild to moderate pain. The only requirement is that the image be vivid, detailed, and involve as many senses as possible.

At the University of Pittsburgh School of Medicine, researchers have classified these mental images into five different categories:

- Pleasant images involving peaceful, pain-free visions.

- Dramatized images where you are part of a dynamic scenario.

- Neutral images, such as recalling the plot of a movie or the rehearsal of plans for the future.

- Environmental images that focus your attention on what you can see in front of you.

- Rhythmic images that come to mind as you sing or count.

Developing the capacity to become engaged in mental images is useful for a number of different purposes. It will help you rehearse desired behavior, relax and release muscle tension, and manage pain.

WEEK 7

HUMAN CONNECTION: The Essence of Health

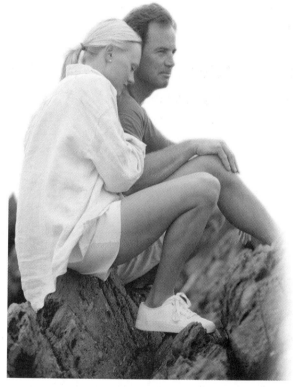

None of us ever accomplishes anything important in isolation. We are relational creatures. This week, you will have the opportunity to explore the importance of human connection.

DAY 43

"Every day she rubs my body, trunk and limbs; her hands knead my back, lift my head, pull my hair–and I feel, intensely, an interdependent fusing together of our bodies and spirits. When she lays hands on my abdomen, pausing, I know that she is praying or meditating the cancer out."

– Donald Hall

We Are All Connected

Studies indicate that people who are married live longer and are healthier than those who are single, separated, widowed, or divorced. Married people are also less likely to get diseases and have a better rate of survival after diagnosis.

The key here isn't necessarily whether or not you're married, but whether you perceive that you have emotional support from family and friends who care about you. Older people who live alone but who perceive themselves surrounded by people who care about them live longer, healthier lives than those who perceive themselves to be emotionally isolated.

We humans are social creatures. We're meant to be in connection with other people. Over and over again, research confirms in quantitative terms the value and benefits of social support.

 ## EAT BETTER: Helping Your Children Eat Well

The best possible way to influence your kids is to be a good role model for them. During the years they are with you, they'll learn many lessons about how to live well and be happy. While most of these lessons will result from what you do right, some of the most important lessons will come from your mistakes.

Daughters, for example, learn a great deal about how to approach food by observing the habits and behavior of their mothers. In fact, eating

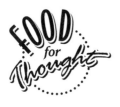

"The words of the
tongue should have
three gatekeepers: Is it
true? Is it kind?
Is it necessary?"

— Arab Proverb

in a way that provides a positive model for her daughter is a good way for a mother to stay on the path herself. It helps to have a few firm guidelines and then to be incredibly flexible on everything else.

Growing children need at least six daily servings of breads and grains, two servings of fruit, three servings of vegetables, three servings of dairy, and at least two servings of protein (meat, poultry, beans, or nuts). These servings can be small if the kids are young.

Try to sneak vegetables into all the dishes you can. Put extra veggies in the pasta, the scrambled eggs, the meatloaf, the soup, the mashed potatoes, the rice, the tossed salad, even the dessert–fat free carrot cake, anyone?

MOVE MORE: Exercise for Your Back

Considering how easy it seems to injure one's back, many doctors no doubt wonder how we manage to walk upright at all. Unfortunately, almost everyone has a bad back story to tell sooner or later. Why not start doing some simple back exercises to strengthen your back today?

The Pelvic Tilt is a fundamental exercise for your lower back that can be done in a few minutes. Lie on your back. As you breathe in, pull in your abdominal muscles as you press your lower back into the floor (by tightening your buttocks and rotating your hips slightly upward). Hold and release.

Doing this exercise for a few minutes every day will be the best prescription your back could ask for.

STRESS LESS: Personal Support

People who belong to gyms or fitness clubs have built-in sources of support for being physically active. It's easy to strike up a conversation with someone in the locker room about the extra mile you walked on the treadmill or your efforts to press another 50 pounds.

Solitary outdoor exercisers don't have such a natural base of support. But people who walk or run, and are serious about it, tend to gravitate to other people like themselves. Some companies sponsor teams to enter local races, and serious amateurs often find themselves discussing workouts around the lunch table.

What kind of social support do you have to be physically active? Maybe the people you live with cheer you on. You may have friends or

DAILY ACTION PLAN

Week_____   Day_____

Date_____   Weight_____

Breakfast	Time:	Protein Grams	Fat Grams	Carbs Grams	Calories
Protein:					
Fruit:					
Grain:					
Beverage:					
Snack	Time:				
Lunch	Time:				
Protein:					
Vegetable:					
Lettuce:					
Grain:					
Fruit:					
Miscellaneous:					
Beverage:					
Snack	Time:				
Dinner	Time:				
Protein:					
Vegetable:					
Lettuce:					
Grain:					
Fruit:					
Miscellaneous:					
Beverage:					
Snack	Time:				
TOTAL					

Today I was able to *Eat Better* by...

_____
_____
_____
_____
_____

Today I was able to *Move More* by...

_____
_____
_____
_____

Today I was able to *Stress Less* by...

_____
_____
_____
_____

Today I feel really great about...

_____
_____
_____
_____

Tomorrow I will focus on...

_____
_____
_____

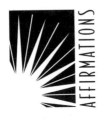

AFFIRMATIONS

"I am a
good friend."

co-workers who like to get out and move just like you. If you enter local races or organized walks, you'll find a community of people you don't even know who have the same interests and fitness goals you do. Above and beyond these personal contacts, reading health and fitness-related newspaper and magazine articles will help support and inspire you.

Support and encouragement to be physically active is everywhere. If it's not at home in your own living room, you can find it out in the world.

DAY 44

"The real key to your influence with me is your example, your actual conduct. Your example flows naturally out of your character, or the kind of person you truly are—not what others say you are or what you may want me to think you are. It is evident in how I actually experience you."
— Stephen R. Covey

How I Experience You

In 1989, David Spiegel and his colleagues at Stanford Medical School demonstrated in a landmark study that women with metastatic breast cancer who were part of an intimate and caring social support group lived twice as long as women who didn't have the support system. This study was especially interesting, because Dr. Spiegel had anticipated the opposite would prove true—that psychological and social support would have no effect on mortality.

This is just one of the many pieces of evidence to show that how we relate to others over the course of our lives significantly affects our health and happiness. Factors that tend to predict health problems are loneliness (social isolation as opposed to the positive implications of chosen solitude), depression, and hostility.

On the other hand, social connection, a feeling of well-being and optimism, and a tolerant, accepting attitude help us stay healthy. Social support during times of stress is especially important in recovery.

EAT BETTER: Order Chinese

Chinese cuisine offers the prospect of delicious and nutritious dining options. But it's also easy to eat enough fat in one meal to *exceed* your allotment for the entire day.

In her book, *The Complete Idiot's Guide to Eating Smart*, Joy Bauer offers the following chart which identifies lower-fat foods that can be substituted for higher-fat options.

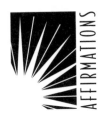

AFFIRMATIONS

"I have harmony
and balance
in my life."

LOWER FAT FOODS	HIGHER FAT FOODS
Hot and sour soup	Egg drop soup
Wonton soup	Egg rolls
Steamed dumplings (vegetable, chicken, and seafood)	Fried dumplings
Stir-fried or steamed chicken and vegetables	Fried wontons
Stir-fried or steamed beef and vegetables	Fried rice
Stir-fried or steamed seafood and vegetables	Egg foo yung
Stir-fried or steamed tofu and vegetables	Cold noodles (with sesame sauce)
Steamed whole fish	Fried fish
Moo-shu vegetables (with pancake rollups)	Moo-shu pork
Steamed brown and white rice	Sweet and sour pork
Fortune cookies	Fried chicken and seafood dishes
Lychee nuts	Seafood (with lobster sauce)
Orange and pineapple slices	Spare ribs
Low-sodium soy sauce, duck sauce, and plum sauce	

MOVE MORE: The Joy of Having a Buddy

Some people look forward to exercise as a solitary experience. They relish the time alone and enjoy the rare opportunity to enjoy their own company without intrusion.

But others like to have company. There are real advantages to having an exercise buddy. The most obvious is that you might not do for yourself what you would do for a friend. Regardless of how much you would disappoint yourself if you didn't keep your commitment to get up and walk at 6:00AM, you would certainly be in trouble if you stood up a friend who waited in the cold for you for a half-hour.

In addition to keeping you honest, a buddy can help you avoid boredom. When your morning walks become as much about conversation as they are about exercise, you'll see what I mean.

A buddy can also help talk you through plateaus or obstacles in your workout program. When you're discouraged, your buddy can say a few

DAILY ACTION PLAN

Week _____ Day _____

Date _____ Weight _____

Breakfast	Time:	Protein Grams	Fat Grams	Carbs Grams	Calories
Protein:					
Fruit:					
Grain:					
Beverage:					
Snack	Time:				
Lunch	Time:				
Protein:					
Vegetable:					
Lettuce:					
Grain:					
Fruit:					
Miscellaneous:					
Beverage:					
Snack	Time:				
Dinner	Time:				
Protein:					
Vegetable:					
Lettuce:					
Grain:					
Fruit:					
Miscellaneous:					
Beverage:					
Snack	Time:				
TOTAL					

Today I was able to *Eat Better* by...

_____

_____

_____

_____

_____

Today I was able to *Move More* by...

_____

_____

_____

_____

Today I was able to *Stress Less* by...

_____

_____

_____

_____

_____

Today I feel really great about...

_____

_____

_____

_____

Tomorrow I will focus on...

_____

_____

_____

_____

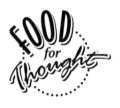

"Treat people as if
they were what
they ought to be
and you help them
to become what they
are capable of being."

— Johann von Goethe

encouraging words or make you laugh, making it that much easier to overcome the obstacles that are slowing you down.

What's more, a buddy can give you a friendly push that's sometimes difficult to give yourself. You might not think of doing that extra lap around the track by yourself, but you may be a bit more willing to give it a try if you have a buddy to do it with.

STRESS LESS: Sharing

You have a lot to give. Everyone does. If you have been paying attention to the blessings in your life, you realize that you have something left over. Sometimes all you have left over is a smile or a pleasant comment to someone you don't know and will never see again. At other times you can share more.

A young friend of mine was once alone in New York City, riding the subway to a job interview. An older woman sitting next to her asked her if she needed help in getting where she was going. By the end of the conversation, this native New Yorker said kindly, "Here's my card, honey. If you ever need a mother in New York, give me a call and I'll be there for you."

What do *you* have to give to someone today?

SUCCESS STORY: Barbra Bercarich

Even though she has maintained a 62 pound weight loss for more than two years, there are times when Barbra Bercarich still does a double-take when she passes a mirror.

"I was overweight for so long that it's taken some time to fully appreciate how different I look and feel today," explains Barbra, 53. "It's hard to believe that's really me in the mirror."

For more years than she cares to count, Barbra struggled with her weight. She tried Weight Watchers, Nutri-System, even the gastric bubble. But every time she lost weight, she regained it.

"When I turned 50, I said to myself, 'This is enough'," she remembers. "I'm 5'7" and I weighed 231 pounds. At that point, I was willing to try anything."

Barbra lost 40 pounds on the Lean for Life program in less than four months, then lost an additional 20 pounds over the following seven months. But Barbra says it's what she *gained* as a result of her weight loss that has changed her life so dramatically.

THEN&NOW

"I'm so much more self-confident and willing to put myself out there now," she says. "My entire attitude and outlook on life is much more open. I was always outgoing, but I was also incredibly self-conscious. Even in the dead of summer, I tried to hide behind my clothes by wearing long pants. One of my friends has a Christmas party every year, and I always made up an excuse why I couldn't go because I never felt truly comfortable in my own skin."

Barbra says her life today feels much more authentic.

"I'm much more comfortable meeting new people and doing new things," she explains. "I feel a sense of confidence and freedom that I really love. I'm much less focused on myself and more open to other people and situations."

While Barbra says she still has an occasional "baby binge", she says her days of devouring junk food are over.

"I was a stress eater, and once I started I couldn't stop," she recalls. "I had no self-control. Zero. I'd stop at a convenience store to buy candy and cookies and would eat it all before I got home. One time I was at my mother's house and ate half of a one-pound bag of Tootsie Rolls. I was embarrassed, so I ran to the store, bought another bag, topped off the jar and then ate the other half-pound on the way home."

Those days, Barbra says, are over.

"I'm not perfect, but I'm so much more conscious today of what I'm eating and why," she says. "And if I do gain a pound or two, I have the tools I need to take care of it before it becomes unmanageable."

DAY 45

"I have no intention of diminishing the power of diet and exercise or, for that matter, of drugs and surgery. There is more scientific evidence now than ever before demonstrating how simple changes in diet and lifestyle may cause significant improvements in health and well-being. As important as these are, I have found that perhaps the most powerful intervention —and the most meaningful for me and for most of the people with whom I work, including staff and patients—is the healing power of love and intimacy, and the emotional and spiritual transformation that often result from these."

— Dean Ornish, M.D.

Positive Connections

There are two other kinds of connections to consider with regard to good health. If you feel that you were loved and cared for by your parents, you are likely to have fewer diseases. If you draw comfort and support from religion, you're also likely to stay healthier.

Some of the positive connections we've been talking about may come to you naturally. You may have grown up in a loving, supportive family. If that's the case, then loving, supportive adult relationships may come naturally to you. If you didn't feel loved and cared about as a child, you may have to work harder to establish nourishing, intimate relationships in your adult life.

It's helpful to remember that your past history is not a certain predictor of your future. You are not sentenced to a future that has already been determined. Your future is truly yours to create. Transformation is a real phenomenon. You *can* change. Once you know what's important, you can acquire the tools to become the person you want to be.

EAT BETTER: Calcium

There is more calcium in your body than any other mineral, with 99% in your bones and 1% in your body fluids. Your body fluids need calcium to regulate normal body functions such as blood pressure, nerve transmission, muscle contraction (including heart beat), clotting of the blood, and the secretion of hormones and digestive enzymes. If there isn't enough calcium in your food, your body fluids will steal from your bones.

In the first 24 years of your life, calcium is important for building bone density. After that, it's essential for maintaining bone density. As you age, your bones gradually lose calcium, especially if you are a postmenopausal woman.

Here, from the NIH Consensus Statement 1994, are the expert recommendations for optimal calcium requirements:

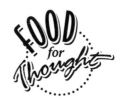

"One cannot have wisdom without living life."

— Dorothy McCall

GROUP	DAILY INTAKE IN MG.
INFANTS	
Birth - 6 months	400
6 months - 1 year	600
CHILDREN	
1 - 5 years	800
6 - 10 years	800 - 1,200
YOUNG ADULTS	
11 - 24 years	1,200 - 1,500
MEN	
25 - 65 years	1,000
Over 65 years	1,500
WOMEN	
25 - 50 years	1,000
Over 50 years (postmenopausal)	
on estrogen	1,000
not on estrogen	1,500
Over 65 years	1,500
Pregnant and nursing	1,200 -1,500

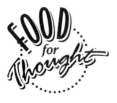

Choose a calcium supplement in the form of calcium carbonate or calcium citrate, and take with it with food. Do not take more than 500 mg. at any one time because more than that can't be absorbed.

Nonfat dairy products, fortified juices and cereals, and canned sardines (with bones) are the biggest suppliers of calcium. Next come canned pink salmon (with bones), and vegetable greens such as collards, turnip greens, kale, and spinach.

MOVE MORE: Thinking About Others

It's surprising how often we feel deep connections to people we've never met. That's one of the *good* things about living in the electronic age and having access to television, newspapers, and computers. We can feel a personal interest in the stories of people we either admire or deplore.

One of the strongest connections is established through athletics or other physical feats. We may not always admire the basketball player known for his trademark slam dunk, but we can relate to the mental and physical discipline he demonstrates when he does it. And our interest and admiration isn't just confined to sports superstars. What about the people who climb Mt. Everest or compete in the Special Olympics? We identify with people who are able to overcome limitations and triumph under pressure.

As you think about your own interests and experience, can you name people with whom you've connected on this level? How did those relationships enhance your life?

STRESS LESS: Walking Meditation

In the Buddhist tradition, there are many different ways to meditate. One of the easiest to learn is the walking meditation. It's like taking a walk, but with a heightened awareness of your surroundings. You slow your pace and open your heart to the sights and sounds along the path.

Thich Nhat Hanh, a Buddhist monk and Nobel Peace Prize nominee, has written about the joys of this simple practice. Here is a quote from his book, *The Long Road Turns to Joy*: "Walking meditation is meditation while walking. We walk slowly, in a relaxed way, keeping a light smile on our lips. When we practice this way, we feel deeply at ease, and our steps are those of the most secure person on Earth. All our

DAILY ACTION PLAN

Week _____   Day _____

Date _____   Weight _____

Breakfast	Time:	Protein Grams	Fat Grams	Carbs Grams	Calories
Protein:					
Fruit:					
Grain:					
Beverage:					
Snack	Time:				
Lunch	Time:				
Protein:					
Vegetable:					
Lettuce:					
Grain:					
Fruit:					
Miscellaneous:					
Beverage:					
Snack	Time:				
Dinner	Time:				
Protein:					
Vegetable:					
Lettuce:					
Grain:					
Fruit:					
Miscellaneous:					
Beverage:					
Snack	Time:				
TOTAL					

Today I was able to *Eat Better* by...

_____
_____
_____
_____

Today I was able to *Move More* by...

_____
_____
_____

Today I was able to *Stress Less* by...

_____
_____
_____
_____
_____

Today I feel really great about...

_____
_____
_____
_____

Tomorrow I will focus on...

_____
_____
_____

sorrows and anxieties drop away, and peace and joy fill our hearts. Anyone can do it. It takes only a little time, a little mindfulness, and the wish to be happy."

Walking can be done in so many different ways. In this, as in everything else, we have choices. Power Walk or Walking Meditation? Every day, the choice is yours.

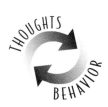

MENTAL FITNESS: The Mirroring Exercise

Looking at yourself in the mirror is a simple act that can become complex when your perceptions have become distorted during weight gain. What you see can be highly subjective. This capacity to see what isn't actually there can work to your advantage when you still want to lose weight. Being able to picture yourself at your ideal weight can help you lose more.

This suggestion comes from Gerald Epstein, M.D., in his book, *Healing Visualizations*: "Imagine seeing yourself in a mirror, seeing yourself thinner there and then seeing yourself enter the mirror and merging with this image. Notice the sensations you experience. Come out of the mirror, stand in front of it again, and push the image out of the mirror to the right with your right hand. Each time you sit down to eat, or several minutes beforehand, see this image you're becoming. You might like to draw this image on a sheet of paper and hang it where you can see it frequently. You might even like to take it with you if you are away from home for long periods of time. Seeing this picture for a moment reinforces your intention."

DAY 46

"Language has the power to transform relationships."
– Harville Hendrix and Helen Hunt

It's How You Say It

We connect with other people through touch. All of us have experienced the life-affirming energy of a hug, but our most important connections often come through the words we speak. When we talk to each other we spin invisible webs that bind us to each other or break the bonds between us.

Think today about how you talk to other people about your weight maintenance program. Do people ask you about your eating and your exercise? And if they do, what do you tell them? What message are you sending about the process of transformation you have undertaken?

When you need help, how do you communicate your need? Do you give off signals, verbal and otherwise, that are more clue-like than clear? Do you hope that people will figure out there is something wrong, or do you let them know exactly what is bothering you?

When you are feeling wonderful about yourself and your accomplishments, how do you convey that?

Think about what message you want to send about your efforts to take care of yourself. A good way to sharpen your understanding of how you seem to others is to imagine that everything you say about your efforts can be overheard by an impressionable young child. In listening to you, what would that child understand about what it means for an adult to make changes in his health?

Remember the power of language, and think about how you can and do use it to impact the lives of the people around you.

EAT BETTER: Alternatives to Eggs

When it comes to making sure you're getting enough protein, eggs can be among your best food choices. They're

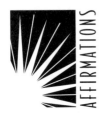

AFFIRMATIONS

"I deserve love."

an excellent source of protein, iron, and vitamin A. Unfortunately, eggs are also relatively high in cholesterol and have five grams of fat in each yolk.

Egg substitutes are a great solution to the "egg problem". They contain all the good stuff without cholesterol and with very little fat. And you can use them in all the ways that you use whole, fresh eggs. There is no way you can tell the difference between whole eggs and egg substitute in a blueberry muffin. Most egg substitutes are sold in the frozen food section of the supermarket.

MOVE MORE: Lessons from Athletes, Part 1

Successful athletes know that they have to spend time preparing for competition. They learn what they need to do to physically, mentally, and emotionally to be in the best possible shape to compete. In other words, they warm-up.

Mental and emotional preparation involves getting yourself in the right frame of mind to accomplish your goals. In order to do that, you need to become highly attuned to your own mental processes. You must come to recognize what it feels like when your thoughts are focused on the task at hand, and learn to recognize when you're distracted. For an athlete, distractions are like death. They can kill a good performance.

You have to develop ways of dealing with distractions so that you're truly free to concentrate on your game. The concentration required for an Olympic high jump is different in some respects from the concentration you'll need over many years to maintain certain habits, but the essence is the same. Keep your goals in mind at all times and never forget that winning requires discipline and desire over the long haul.

STRESS LESS: The Love Note

In five minutes, you can strengthen the bond between yourself and someone you love by writing a "love note". Reading a note from someone who loves you is magical. Your sagging spirits are buoyed up, your work load is lightened, and you think about how much you love the writer.

There are different kinds of love notes. There is the kind of note a mother tucks into her child's lunch box on the first day of school. There's the kind of note a woman sends to her sister after surgery. There is the

DAILY ACTION PLAN

Week _____ Day _____

Date _____ Weight _____

Breakfast	Time:	Protein Grams	Fat Grams	Carbs Grams	Calories
Protein:					
Fruit:					
Grain:					
Beverage:					
Snack	Time:				
Lunch	Time:				
Protein:					
Vegetable:					
Lettuce:					
Grain:					
Fruit:					
Miscellaneous:					
Beverage:					
Snack	Time:				
Dinner	Time:				
Protein:					
Vegetable:					
Lettuce:					
Grain:					
Fruit:					
Miscellaneous:					
Beverage:					
Snack	Time:				
TOTAL					

Today I was able to *Eat Better* by...

_____

_____

_____

_____

Today I was able to *Move More* by...

_____

_____

_____

_____

Today I was able to *Stress Less* by...

_____

_____

_____

_____

Today I feel really great about...

_____

_____

_____

_____

Tomorrow I will focus on...

_____

_____

_____

_____

kind of note a husband leaves for his wife in anticipation of a passionate evening, and the kind a co-worker writes to another co-worker who's struggling through a tough time.

When you write a "love note", you'll almost feel as though you're the recipient because the good feelings that result will contribute to a healthier you. You might even try writing a love note to yourself!

"There is a certain blend of courage, integrity, character, and principle which has no satisfactory dictionary name but has been called different things at different times in different countries. Our American name for it is 'guts'."

– Louis Adamic

Guts

Whether you call it guts, gumption, determination, tenacity, or courage, the capacity to identify a goal and achieve it is definitely an advantage in achieving successful weight maintenance. To set a course and follow it over both the rough and the smooth terrain of your life journey requires a blend of courage, integrity, and character.

Can you think of a time in recent weeks when you did something you thought took guts? I'm not talking about the kind of guts it takes to pull a drowning man out of a river or stand up for a principle in the face of vocal opposition. I'm talking about a quieter, more personal brand of courage.

You'll likely think of something you did within a social context. You fixed your brother's favorite Italian dinner, and still stayed on your eating plan. You spoke up when your boorish co-worker commented on what you were eating for lunch. You signed up for an aerobics class.

Courage in the face of big challenges is important. But courage in dealing with the small, everyday issues that make up most of our lives is also the mark of who you are as a person.

 ## EAT BETTER: Grocery Shopping

It's very hard to eat nutritiously at home if you don't have the food you need to stay on your plan. It's even harder if you have tempting high fat options within easy reach. If you don't have a good, enriched cereal available, you're more likely to resort to peanut butter on toast.

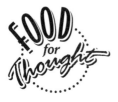

"The weak can never forgive. Forgiveness is the attribute of the strong."

— Mahatma Gandhi

The key to a well-stocked maintenance food pantry is smart grocery shopping. And the key to smart grocery shopping is a good list. In fact, you might consider typing a sample list and making copies so you have one available every time you go shopping. Your list might include categories with enough space under each one to write in specific items. The following categories work well for most people:

- Grains
- Dairy
- Protein
- Vegetables
- Fruits
- Beverages

- Prepared Foods (frozen)
- Prepared Foods (canned)
- Snacks
- Condiments
- Fats
- Non-Food Personal Items

Add to this list anything you can think of, and then use it. It will help make a difference in how you shop and how you eat!

MOVE MORE: Lessons for Athletes, Part 2

Sports psychologists and others who study peak performance in athletes boil down their complex findings into a rather simple statement: "Peak performance is characterized by high-energy intensity and a sense of inner calmness."

This may sound like a contradiction. How can someone be both intense and calm at the same time? Calmness refers to a state of mental relaxation and implies a sense of being in control, feeling optimistic, and having all the time you need to do what you have to do. These feelings aren't at all the opposite of high energy. In fact, when you think about it, you'll realize that you often feel your most energetic when you are calm, optimistic, and unhurried.

What does this mean to you? For one thing, it means you can be aware that you function best when you've achieved a state of high energy and inner calm, and you can do those things that tend to promote these characteristics.

It might be useful to write down a list of things you can do in your life to achieve and maintain high energy and inner calm. Here's a hint: Many of the answers are featured in this book.

DAILY ACTION PLAN

Week _____   Day _____

Date _____   Weight _____

Breakfast	Time:	Protein Grams	Fat Grams	Carbs Grams	Calories
Protein:					
Fruit:					
Grain:					
Beverage:					
Snack	Time:				
Lunch	Time:				
Protein:					
Vegetable:					
Lettuce:					
Grain:					
Fruit:					
Miscellaneous:					
Beverage:					
Snack	Time:				
Dinner	Time:				
Protein:					
Vegetable:					
Lettuce:					
Grain:					
Fruit:					
Miscellaneous:					
Beverage:					
Snack	Time:				
TOTAL					

Today I was able to *Eat Better* by...

_____
_____
_____
_____
_____

Today I was able to *Move More* by...

_____
_____
_____
_____

Today I was able to *Stress Less* by...

_____
_____
_____
_____

Today I feel really great about...

_____
_____
_____
_____

Tomorrow I will focus on...

_____
_____
_____

STRESS LESS: The Virtues of "Giving In"

Some people absolutely must have the last word. Whether you're a "last worder" or you simply live with, work with, or know someone who is, you can probably see the humor in the "last word" compulsion. The conflict is finally resolved amicably, a few moments of silence puts the seal on your agreement, and then one of you suddenly adds, "OK, but I still think. . ."

If you can relate to this, you might consider making a decision right now to approach the next disagreement a little differently. The next time your temperature rises and find yourself arguing with someone, try making your point and then stopping. Instead of persisting, say, "OK. I see your point. Maybe you're right."

In other words, try giving up and giving in. The value for you is to experience what it's like to give up the need to be right, the need to persuade, and the need to control. It's a symbolic act that says, "I don't know everything. I can't control everything. Other people see it differently and that's all right with me."

Try it. See what happens.

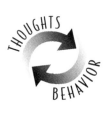

MENTAL FITNESS : Avoidance–Making It Easier for Yourself

Who says you must always step up to the challenge or face all obstacles head-on? Especially during the early months of maintenance, it may be necessary to adopt a more realistic stance toward the people and places that trigger old behavior.

Certain foods, people, and situations may make you want to revert to being an overfed slug. It's wise to be aware of what these triggers are and avoid them. Don't buy the donuts "for the kids"; don't spend the entire weekend with your old party friends; don't spend your vacation on a cruise ship instead of hiking in the Rockies.

Learning how to better control your environment is just as important as learning how to influence your thoughts and feelings.

DAY 48

"Be kind, for everyone you meet is fighting a hard battle."
– Plato

Kindness: The Glue of Human Connection

Kindness. It sounds like such an old-fashioned word. It conjures up images of another age–old women being kind to distraught youngsters, nurses being kind to wounded soldiers.

Perhaps it's time to reintroduce the concept. What I mean by kindness is gentleness, tolerance, caring, and a desire to help others. These are noble virtues in the realm of human relations. A bigger dose of ordinary kindness would make the world a better place.

But we want to emphasize how important it is to be kind *inside* your own skin; to turn the warm light of kindness on within yourself. To be gentle with yourself. To develop a tolerance for your own human frailties. To care about the hidden and wounded parts of you that are doing the best they can. To learn how to help yourself move forward, instead of punishing yourself. A bigger dose of kindness *inside* would also make your inner world a better place.

EAT BETTER: Ideas for Healthy Snacks

As you know, snacks are the "bread and butter" of your food plan. Having good snacking options available when you need them is essential. Here are some suggestions:

- protein drinks

- high protein nutritional bars

- air-popped popcorn

- pretzels

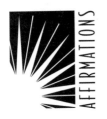

"I am worthy of love and respect."

- graham crackers and skim milk

- fig bars and skim milk

- sliced fruit

- shredded wheat (dry)

- low fat trail mix

- frozen fruit bars

- frozen yogurt pops

- carrots and celery with nonfat ranch dressing

- yogurt and low fat granola

You can make it a habit to collect good snacking ideas from other people. Notice what other health-conscious, trim people choose for snacks, and see if that makes sense for you.

MOVE MORE: Lessons from Athletes, Part 3

Some people function at their best in stressful situations. Others react to the mildest difficulties by falling apart and totally "stressing out".

It's important to observe this disparity between external stressors and internal reactions to stress, because it provides us with important information about peak performance.

High level athletes know that stress results from one's response to the environment more than from the environment itself. The important thing is not what is happening, but how you *respond* to what is happening.

You can see how important attitude is. People who are resilient and have strong coping skills generally possess certain qualities:

- They believe they can influence events around them and act as though what they do matters.

- They commit to action instead of becoming passive.

- They believe that change and challenge are natural, rather than disruptive, unusual occurrences.

DAILY ACTION PLAN

Week _____   Day _____

Date _____   Weight _____

Breakfast Time:	Protein Grams	Fat Grams	Carbs Grams	Calories
Protein:				
Fruit:				
Grain:				
Beverage:				
Snack Time:				
Lunch Time:				
Protein:				
Vegetable:				
Lettuce:				
Grain:				
Fruit:				
Miscellaneous:				
Beverage:				
Snack Time:				
Dinner Time:				
Protein:				
Vegetable:				
Lettuce:				
Grain:				
Fruit:				
Miscellaneous:				
Beverage:				
Snack Time:				
TOTAL				

Today I was able to *Eat Better* by...

_____

_____

_____

_____

Today I was able to *Move More* by...

_____

_____

_____

_____

Today I was able to *Stress Less* by...

_____

_____

_____

_____

Today I feel really great about...

_____

_____

_____

_____

Tomorrow I will focus on...

_____

_____

_____

_____

You don't have to be a world-class athlete or a top-level executive to benefit from these insights. You can begin managing stress more effectively by adopting and applying some of these attitudes in your own life.

STRESS LESS: Breathing Stress Breaks

We've already discussed the restorative power of breathing. Here are some effortless strategies for including more cleansing breaths in your daily routine:

- Whenever you stop for a red light, take a deep breath. As you exhale, envision yourself easing into a warm bath. Relax and let go.

- Just before you answer the phone, take a deep breath and relax as you breathe out.

- Just before you turn on your computer or turn it off, take the same kind of cleansing breath.

- Do the same every time you get up from your chair, or sit back down again.

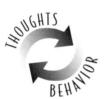

MENTAL FITNESS: Rehearsing Connection

This mental training session will help you rehearse a situation with another person that you anticipate may be stressful. Begin by relaxing, then generate imagery that lets you play the scene in a way that is positive.

Find a comfortable place where you can be alone for about ten minutes. Close your eyes and breath in and out deeply for five breaths. With each breathing in take in positive energy, and with each breathing out let go of muscle tension that you don't need.

Let yourself visualize the place where your expected encounter will take place. Look around and see what the place looks like. Let yourself feel comfortable at being there. Next, let yourself see the person you are going to meet. Linger over the details of how he or she looks and sounds. Then, let yourself experience the encounter going well: conflicts are resolved, distrust dissolves, and anger gets expressed in a healthy way. Let yourself say what you want to say and really listen to what the other person has to say. Experience how you want to feel during the encounter and after. Give yourself permission to feel pleased at the conclusion.

You might want to use mental rehearsal several times to prepare for occasions that are important to you. You will find that your positive expectations of the event will profoundly influence your manner and, therefore, the event itself.

Your Turn.

Living With Gratitude

Today I live my life with an attitude of gratitude.

Today I am grateful for_____

_____

_____

_____

_____

_____

_____

_____

_____

_____

_____

_____

DAY 49

"There are two cornerstone ideas that appear again and again in most spiritual writings on relationships. On the one hand, there is the notion that we are all one. . . On the other hand, there is the notion that each of us is whole, complete, and perfect–exactly as we are."

– Rick Fields

Exactly As I Am

Imagine what it would feel like to accept yourself exactly as you are at this moment, without reservation, without wishing anything about your body or your life were different. To know and feel that you are just fine the way you are right now is a remarkable, liberating joy that too few of us allow ourselves to ever experience.

Wherever you are in your life journey, you've done what you needed to do to survive. Along the way, you've even thrived and triumphed at some of what you've attempted. You've struggled, as we all have. If your body is still bigger or not in as a good a shape as you'd like, you simply aren't finished learning yet. If you still aren't as active as you'd like, you have more adventures ahead of you.

We all know that life is a process, but what we often forget is that we're just fine at every step along the way. There is no finish line. There is only today. So practice self-acceptance and even self-appreciation. When you do, you'll find it easier to accept and appreciate other people, too.

 ### EAT BETTER: Fast Food

Fast food is the American way of life. It's convenient, cheap, and readily available no matter where you go. Fortunately, you have more low fat choices at fast food restaurants than you did a decade ago. Just remember that when placing your order at the drive-thru window, you'll do best to avoid anything that's fried or comes with "special sauce" or cheese. Stick with dishes that are as plain and simple as possible, such as:

- Veggie burgers (no mayo)

- Turkey sandwiches (no mayo)

- Chicken fajitas

- Bean burritos (no cheese)

- Baked potatoes (no butter; nonfat sour cream; soy-based bacon bits)

- Vegetarian chili

- Grilled or steamed vegetables

- Fresh fruit

- Green salads with no dressing or low fat dressing

- Pancakes (no butter)

- Bagel and jelly

- Grilled chicken sandwich (no mayo or sauce)

If other people want to stop for a quick burger, you can eat right along with them. Just be conscious of your choices. One fast food meal can contain more fat, carbohydrates, and calories than you need for an entire day.

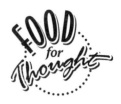

"To love oneself is the beginning of a lifelong romance."

— Oscar Wilde

MOVE MORE: Lessons from Athletes, Part 4

Here's a simple imaging technique that many successful athletes use to enhance their performance. Choose an animal that has the characteristics you want to acquire. Visualize that animal in all its athletic grace and beauty, and experience yourself becoming that animal whenever you are in a situation that calls for it.

We know one successful maintainer who imagines herself as a cheetah. She envies and emulates the sleek power of this beautiful cat. We know another woman who has chosen a gazelle, and yet another who identifies with a horse. When you think about these choices, each person is expressing a desire for a different strength.

During your next relaxation/visualization, take three deep breaths, relax your body, and let yourself visualize the animal you want to be. Choose an animal who possesses the qualities you need in order to accomplish your maintenance goals. Imagine as many details of color, form, and movement as you can.

After the visualization session, practice calling up the image of your animal as often as you can until it becomes second nature. As you re-experience your animal, you will integrate its qualities into yourself a little more every day.

STRESS LESS: I Need You

"I need you."

These are golden words to most people. Most of us want to be needed. We want the people we care about to ask us for help and solace when they need it.

The next time you're feeling isolated or distressed, reach out to someone. Pick up the phone and call a friend or family member. You don't have to tell them more than you want. Just let them know that you need to talk. Something like this: "Hi. It's me. I'm feeling kind of blah, so I thought I'd give you a call. Do you have time for me to talk a little bit. I just need someone to listen. Is that OK?"

Imagine a friend approaching you in this way. You'd be glad to listen, wouldn't you? So will your friends.

DAILY ACTION PLAN

Week _____   Day _____

Date _____   Weight _____

Breakfast	Time:	Protein Grams	Fat Grams	Carbs Grams	Calories
Protein:					
Fruit:					
Grain:					
Beverage:					
Snack	Time:				
Lunch	Time:				
Protein:					
Vegetable:					
Lettuce:					
Grain:					
Fruit:					
Miscellaneous:					
Beverage:					
Snack	Time:				
Dinner	Time:				
Protein:					
Vegetable:					
Lettuce:					
Grain:					
Fruit:					
Miscellaneous:					
Beverage:					
Snack	Time:				
TOTAL					

Today I was able to *Eat Better* by...

_____

_____

_____

_____

Today I was able to *Move More* by...

_____

_____

_____

_____

Today I was able to *Stress Less* by...

_____

_____

_____

_____

Today I feel really great about...

_____

_____

_____

Tomorrow I will focus on...

_____

_____

_____

WEEK 8

COMMITMENT: The Energy to Keep Going

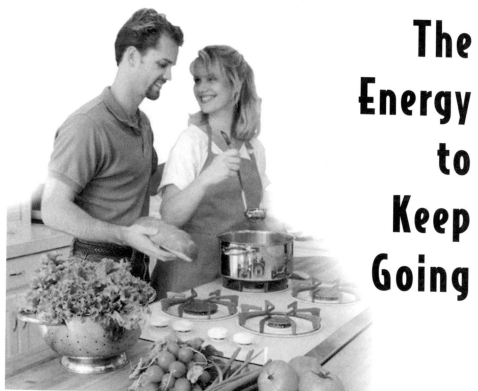

As a lifelong maintainer, you will learn what you need to do to keep yourself going in the right direction. Your progress will be part determination and part enthusiasm. During this last week of the program, you'll appreciate all of the factors we've discussed so far, and continue developing a way of living that will serve you well for the rest of your life.

"So the inner passion of a strong emotional commitment is a facilitating, liberating, and immensely productive force in the life of any individual. With it we conquer challenges; without it we stumble. With it we are willing to take risks when needed; without it we just play it safe. With it we strive for excellence; without it we settle for much, much less."

– *Tom Morris*

The Inner Passion of Strong Emotional Commitment

Your desire to gain greater control over your life grew from a spark into a flame. Somewhere along the line, there was a moment when you decided to do things differently. You couldn't have known at the beginning what that would mean, yet you instinctively knew you wanted more out of life than you were getting. You decided to do whatever was necessary to change.

In order to be where you are now, you fanned that spark into a strong emotional commitment. You've experienced what a strong emotional commitment feels like, and where it can lead you. In this case, it has lead to greater awareness in every aspect of your life. A simple desire to weigh less has ultimately become a desire to live more fully.

You can use what you've learned about yourself throughout this process and apply it to other areas of your life. Is there something you've always wanted to accomplish but have never felt confident enough to pursue? Is there a spark of interest that you want to fan into a flame? If there is, go for it. What are you waiting for?

EAT BETTER: A Passion for Eating

Since you're in the last week of this program, it's a good time to take stock of where you are in relation to food. How have your eating habits and your feelings about

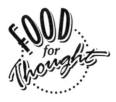

"You don't get to choose how you're going to die, or when. You can only decide how you're going to live. Now."

— Joan Baez

food changed over the preceding weeks? Are you getting closer to the kind of relationship with food you want to have?

Ideally, you'll now feel enough in control to pick and choose what you eat and to eat what you've chosen with great gusto. Your friend may be having three-cheese lasagna, but his enthusiasm for his dish won't be any greater than your enthusiasm for your plate of grilled halibut with fresh lemon.

Ideally, you've learned how to plan ahead. You know what works for breakfast, lunch, dinner, and snacks, and you have easy access to your choices. They're available when you want (or need) them.

Ideally, you're able to treat yourself to dishes that aren't part of your regular food plan. And when you do indulge, you know how to make adjustments in eating and exercise to compensate for the extra fat and calories you've consumed.

You may not have reached your ideal yet. That's why maintenance is a life-time endeavor. But wherever you are right now, take the time to feel good about how far you've come. Remember back to when you were still overweight and struggling every day.

Keep working at it. The benefits you've gained from what you've already done are priceless.

MOVE MORE: Ten Reasons to Get Moving!

Our bodies were meant to move. Whenever you're feeling sluggish or lazy, remember these ten reasons why:

1. Moving brings oxygen to each and every cell in your body, including your brain. An oxygenated brain is an alert brain.

2. Moving increases your energy level, making you feel less tired and able to do more work.

3. Moving increases cardiorespiratory fitness and reduces disease risk.

4. Moving improves your circulation; your reflexes become quicker and your joints move through their whole range of motion.

5. Moving helps you sleep better at night.

6. Moving gives you healthy, glowing skin.

7. Moving stimulates your digestion, yet controls your appetite.

8. Moving tones your muscles, making you appear trimmer.

9. Moving boosts your self-confidence.

10. *Moving helps you maintain your weight!*

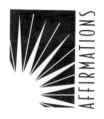

 ## STRESS LESS: Time to Write in Your Journal

Enthusiasm and passion for doing something that's important to you offers good journaling opportunities. Just as it's helpful (and even transforming) to write regularly about your blessings, writing about people, places, and experiences can remind you of the many joys in your life. What do you love to do? What experiences have you had that make your heart sing and your temperature rise?

Take a few moments to allow memories to surface. Choose two events or activities that you recall most vividly and fondly. Close your eyes and allow yourself to visualize each of them fully in your imagination. Recreate these special moments in your mind. Then write about them, trying to capture the essence of what makes them so memorable for you.

We asked a group of Lindora patients to talk about their passions, and here are a few of their responses:

- "I'm ecstatic when I am singing in the Symphonic Choir. Nothing else makes me so happy."

- "I love the sense of tranquility, solitude, and inner peace I experience whenever I go backpacking."

- "Since I'm always on the run, what I really adore more than anything is sitting in my window seat on a rainy day, reading a good book with my cat curled up in my lap."

- "I feel most passionate and alive when I'm teaching adults to read through a literacy program where I volunteer every Saturday morning."

Enthusiasm is the energy that fuels your life. Duty and responsibility are important and also provide fuel, but enthusiasm helps you reach beyond what you've done in the past to attain new heights and to experience life in remarkably rich new ways.

"I am enjoying the results of my efforts and energy."

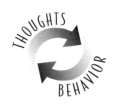

MENTAL FITNESS: Maintenance and Enjoyment

Overweight people often feel burdened by duties and obligations to other people. In symbolic terms, they carry the weight of heavy expectations around with them wherever they go. Sometimes food is the one thing they can rely on to provide pleasure and consolation.

These same people, when they decide to lose weight, make a commitment to broaden the scope of their enjoyment. They want to find more pleasure, satisfaction, fulfillment, and fun in their lives. They become convinced there is more to life than the eternal round of sleeping, working, eating, and making other people happy.

As their weight decreases, their enjoyment in life inevitably increases. Living leaner means having more energy and more confidence to do the things they've always wanted to do. Weight loss helps facilitate these changes, and these changes encourage more weight loss. The spiral cycles upward toward health instead of downward toward illness.

Maintaining weight loss means never having to fight the same battles or face the same demons as before. Physical and emotional energy is freed for pursuing life goals instead of struggling with weight. Imagine the freedom of never having to lose weight again! It can be yours.

SUCCESS STORY: Dr. Tari Lennon

Have you ever gone to the gym and experienced a sudden wave of sensory overload? There's a flurry of activity everywhere you look. Bodies–lots of bodies–are moving fast and in every possible direction. The music from your Walkman competes with the music that blares over the gym's stereo system.

Tari Lennon has been there, and she didn't like it. Determined to become more fit and active after losing 70 pounds on her Lean for Life program two years ago, the 62-year-old pastor and clinical psychologist joined a gym after several friends persuaded her to go with them for workouts.

"At first, I thought the 'buddy system' would be a terrific incentive to stick to a regular schedule," says Tari. "But what dawned on me rather quickly is the simple fact that my life is already overly structured and full of people and time commitments. Another commitment on my calendar isn't what I needed. My challenge was finding time–*making* time–to take of myself, to get quiet, and to enjoy solitude."

THEN&NOW

That's exactly what she's done. She no longer spends her exercise time at the gym. Instead, she walks early in the morning on a quiet hillside path near her home with her dogs, Whitman and Emily. When she uses her treadmill at home, she usually makes a point to do nothing else while walking.

"I find that quiet time spent alone is enormously healthy and valuable," she says. "When I do a half-hour on the treadmill with no TV or stereo or magazine to distract my attention and occupy my time, I'm much more aware of my thoughts, feelings, and physical sensations. It's a sort of altered state in which I find myself able to achieve a clarity of thought, a sense of balance and an inner tranquility that's impossible to achieve when I'm with other people or reacting to outside stimulation."

Tari says that since deciding to make physical activity a greater priority in her life, she finds there's a direct connection between her elevated energy and how she feels about herself.

"When I go too long without physical activity, I'm sluggish and more likely to feel negative and depressed," she explains. "Knowing that, I do whatever I can to build physical activity into my day. Even when I can only squeeze in 15 minutes on the treadmill, I still experience a sense of accomplishment in doing it. For me, losing weight–and maintaining the success I've achieved–is about reclaiming a sense of control and being in the best physical place I can be at this age and stage of my life. And at this stage in my life, doing what works and feels good for me whenever I can is an important part of my spiritual journey."

DAILY ACTION PLAN

Week _____   Day _____

Date _____   Weight _____

Breakfast Time:	Protein Grams	Fat Grams	Carbs Grams	Calories
Protein:				
Fruit:				
Grain:				
Beverage:				
Snack Time:				
Lunch Time:				
Protein:				
Vegetable:				
Lettuce:				
Grain:				
Fruit:				
Miscellaneous:				
Beverage:				
Snack Time:				
Dinner Time:				
Protein:				
Vegetable:				
Lettuce:				
Grain:				
Fruit:				
Miscellaneous:				
Beverage:				
Snack Time:				
TOTAL				

Today I was able to *Eat Better* by...

_____
_____
_____
_____

Today I was able to *Move More* by...

_____
_____
_____
_____

Today I was able to *Stress Less* by...

_____
_____
_____
_____
_____

Today I feel really great about...

_____
_____
_____
_____

Tomorrow I will focus on...

_____
_____
_____
_____

DAY 51

"There were times when I could not afford to sacrifice the bloom of the present moment to any work, whether of the head or hand. I love a broad margin to my life. Sometimes, in a summer morning, having taken my accustomed bath, I sat in my sunny doorway from sunrise till noon, rapt in a reverie, midst the pines and hickories and sumacs, in undisturbed solitude and stillness, while the birds sang around or flitted noiseless through the house, until by the sun falling in at my west window, or the noise of some traveler's wagon on the distant highway, I was reminded of the lapse of time."

– Henry David Thoreau

The Bloom of the Present Moment

Thoreau's words are like a letter from the past, a message from another time.

He speaks of a world that permits him a rapt reverie lasting half the day. But our lives today are different. Most of us feel compelled to spend every last minute doing *something*–sometimes so many "somethings" that we lose count of them all.

But does it *have* to be this way? Let's pause for a minute and consider how many of our limitations are real and how many are self-imposed, composed of half-true assumptions about what we *should* be doing and what life is *supposed to be* like. Most of these assumptions are about time. We don't have enough of it. If we only had more, we'd be better people, and we'd be happier.

The truth is that we have the same number of hours in a day as Thoreau did. It's true that our modern lives are radically different in many ways, but it's worth stopping to examine the assumption that we never have time to watch the setting sun or the birds in the trees. This is "soul time". We need it in the same measure that Thoreau needed it, and we ignore these needs at our peril.

EAT BETTER: What If You're Drinking Your Fruit?

Drinking fruit juice isn't quite as nutritious as eating fresh fruit because you miss out on the fiber, but it's still a whole lot better than drinking a cola. Here's a comparison:

8 OUNCES OF ORANGE JUICE	8 OUNCES OF COLA
110 calories	100 calories
26 grams of carbohydrate	26 grams of carbohydrate
0 fat	0 fat
25 grams of sugar	26 grams of sugar
120% vitamin C	0% vitamin C
12% potassium	0% potassium
20% folic acid	0% folic acid

Fruit juice is good, and so is fresh water. It contains no sugar, no calories, and no caffeine!

MOVE MORE: What Successful Maintainers Say About Exercise

People who have exercised over a period of years have plenty of positive things to say about the role it plays in their lives.

"Exercise is as much a part of my life as eating or sleeping." Many long-time exercisers have incorporated exercise into their daily routines so completely that it becomes invisible. They don't have to ask themselves whether or not they're going to get on the bike or walk the track that day because the answer is always "yes."

"My body is so finely tuned now that if I miss even two days of exercise, I can really feel a difference." It takes a awhile to realize how your daily exercise session affects your appetite, your mood, and your energy level, but when you do figure it out, you come to value–and rely on–the benefits.

"When I read an article in a magazine or see a program on TV about white water rafting, or bicycling from Portland to San Francisco for a fundraiser, I think to myself, 'I could do that.'" When you've met physical challenges and watched yourself get better at something over time, you become confident in your ability to meet new challenges. You can have a dream and immediately start working toward it . Your dreams don't stall because you aren't physically able to realize them.

"I can't imagine going back." This comment says it all.

STRESS LESS: Patience

Think of this as an exercise in developing character and patience. It goes like this: Whenever the time is right, introduce a subject that you know a friend or family member has strong feelings about. Politics is always a surefire conversation starter!

Then listen with interest while the other person talks. If you have strong feelings on the subject, so much the better. But don't share them. Instead, practice giving the other person your undivided attention. Whether you agree or disagree doesn't matter. What matters is that you practice being present in the moment and letting the other person know you are hearing what they say.

We talked earlier about the healing benefits that result from really listening to another person–benefits not only for you, but for the person who feels they are truly being heard. Now you can add character building to the list of reasons to practice good listening skills!

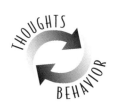

MENTAL FITNESS: Increasing Your Creativity

In his book, *Creativity*, Mihaly Csikszentmihalyi summarizes what he's learned from highly creative people about how they make their day-to-day experience of living more vivid, enjoyable, and rewarding. Here, briefly, are some of his ideas:

CURIOSITY AND INTEREST.

- Try to be surprised by something every day.

- Try to surprise at least one person every day.

DAILY ACTION PLAN

Week _____   Day _____

Date _____   Weight _____

Breakfast	Time:	Protein Grams	Fat Grams	Carbs Grams	Calories
Protein:					
Fruit:					
Grain:					
Beverage:					
Snack	Time:				
Lunch	Time:				
Protein:					
Vegetable:					
Lettuce:					
Grain:					
Fruit:					
Miscellaneous:					
Beverage:					
Snack	Time:				
Dinner	Time:				
Protein:					
Vegetable:					
Lettuce:					
Grain:					
Fruit:					
Miscellaneous:					
Beverage:					
Snack	Time:				
TOTAL					

Today I was able to *Eat Better* by...

_____
_____
_____
_____
_____

Today I was able to *Move More* by...

_____
_____
_____
_____

Today I was able to *Stress Less* by...

_____
_____
_____
_____
_____

Today I feel really great about...

_____
_____
_____
_____

Tomorrow I will focus on...

_____
_____
_____
_____

- Write down each day what surprised you and how you surprised others.

- When something strikes a spark of interest, follow it.

CULTIVATING "FLOW" IN EVERYDAY LIFE.

- Wake up in the morning with a specific goal to look forward to.

- If you do something well, it becomes enjoyable.

- To keep enjoying something, you need to increase its complexity.

HABITS OF STRENGTH.

- Take charge of your schedule.

- Make time for reflection and relaxation.

- Shape your space.

- Find out what you like and what you hate about life.

- Start doing more of what you love and less of what you hate.

These ideas are distilled from years of interviews with exceptional people. They are simple to understand but not always simple to do. Take your time reading the list, and think about how you might use each suggestion.

In a couple of days, we'll look at more of Csikszentmihalyi's suggestions for living life with greater purpose and passion.

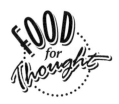

"Patience is a particular requirement. Without it, you can destroy in an hour what it might take you weeks to repair."

— Charlie W. Shedd

DAY 52

"Each of us is born with two contradictory sets of instructions: a conservative tendency, made up of instincts for self-preservation, self-aggrandizement, and saving energy, and an expansive tendency made up of instincts for exploring, for enjoying novelty and risk–the curiosity that leads to creativity belongs to this set."

– Mihaly Csikszentmihalyi

Contradictions

We all know how it feels to experience contradictory, conflicting values. There is a part of us that wants to do one thing and another that wants the opposite. We want that piece of chocolate cake/we don't want that piece of chocolate cake. We want to start that exercise class/we don't want to start that exercise class. We want to sleep in/we want to get an early start on the day.

Confusing? Of course, but it's a fact of life that few human beings are totally consistent. But rather than seeing this as a problem, consider it a challenge.

Reconciling within yourself (or at least containing within yourself) contradictory elements creates an opportunity for creativity. You generate more options and see more connections than otherwise.

So next time you're upset by those warring voices within, remember that this kind of complexity helps you grow.

EAT BETTER: "Just a Taste"

One way you'll know when you are in control of your eating instead of being controlled *by* your eating is when you can have a taste of something you love and leave it at that. You can have a small piece of pie and be thrilled. You can have one cookie (or one potato chip, for that matter) and not need to eat the whole bag. You become an artist, picking and choosing the colors and tastes that make your experience complete.

MOVE MORE: 10,000 Steps

As you know, we at Lindora are great believers in counting steps. The pedometer is such an easy way to keep track of how active you are. At Lindora, 10,000 steps a day is a goal. Research from Japan demonstrates that women who average less than 7,500 steps a day begin to accumulate intra-abdominal fat, the type of fat that is a factor in diabetes and diseases of the heart. We know that exercise is important. It burns calories and builds muscles. The more muscles you have, the more calories you'll burn–even when sleeping! Exercise helps people maintain their weight. Successful maintainers in the National Weight Loss Registry walked an average of 28 miles per week. That averages four miles a day, which equals about 10,000 steps per day! So step it up!

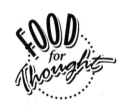

"The invariable mark of wisdom is to see the miraculous in the common."

— Ralph Waldo Emerson

STRESS LESS: Shyness

You'd be surprised at how many people think of themselves as shy. They're uncomfortable being the center of attention, and they feel like the center a lot of the time. Although many children grow out of shyness to become more socially comfortable, many highly-functioning adults continue to feel uneasy in social situations.

One recommendation psychologists make for overcoming shyness is to gradually desensitize yourself. Expose yourself in a controlled way to what you are afraid of. In the case of shyness, make it a point to have contact with as many people as you can throughout the day.

The idea is that you practice your social skills in whatever ways present themselves. You speak in front of your parents' group; you offer to host a foreign exchange student; you chair the committee meeting. It's not that practice necessarily makes it easier (although it usually does), but you gain the satisfaction of knowing that you can function well in a social setting, no matter what your internal comfort level.

DAILY ACTION PLAN

Week _____ Day _____

Date _____ Weight _____

Breakfast Time:	Protein Grams	Fat Grams	Carbs Grams	Calories
Protein:				
Fruit:				
Grain:				
Beverage:				
Snack Time:				
Lunch Time:				
Protein:				
Vegetable:				
Lettuce:				
Grain:				
Fruit:				
Miscellaneous:				
Beverage:				
Snack Time:				
Dinner Time:				
Protein:				
Vegetable:				
Lettuce:				
Grain:				
Fruit:				
Miscellaneous:				
Beverage:				
Snack Time:				
TOTAL				

Today I was able to *Eat Better* by...

_____

_____

_____

_____

Today I was able to *Move More* by...

_____

_____

_____

_____

Today I was able to *Stress Less* by...

_____

_____

_____

_____

Today I feel really great about...

_____

_____

_____

_____

Tomorrow I will focus on...

_____

_____

_____

_____

DAY 53

"The point here is simply that it is useful at times to admit to yourself that you don't know your way and to be open to help from unexpected places. Doing this makes available to you inner and outer energies and allies that arise out of your own soulfulness and selflessness."

– Jon Kabat-Zinn

Knowing Your Way

There are times when we lose our way. This fact seems to be built into the human development blueprint. Things go along fine for some time, and then for either external or internal reasons, they're suddenly not fine anymore. What we've been doing no longer works or feels worth doing.

While it doesn't seem like it at the time, the times when we seem to lose our way are gifts. They give us an opportunity to explore what we're doing and why, to examine our value systems and operating principles. In a manner of speaking, the tough times require us to tend to our internal gardens so that new seeds can be planted and new goals and dreams can grow.

This can happen, however, only if we're willing to dig deeply enough in the garden. We don't always have to know what row we're planting, but its very helpful to know which direction we're headed. Having a purpose for your life gives you enthusiasm, passion, creativity–all the qualities we've been talking about over the past seven weeks.

When your purpose changes (as it will) or you lose it (which you will), remember that it's important to focus on finding it again. When your children grow up and leave home, you may need to evaluate and redefine your purpose in life. The same is true for any major life change, as well as for the smaller, individual life changes known only to you.

Ask yourself right now what your purpose in life is. Why are you here? If you're not sure, then you've just stumbled on an opportunity to take a major step forward by seeking the answer.

EAT BETTER: How Far You've Come

Close your eyes and recall what your eating was like yesterday. Can you remember what you ate throughout the day? What does your mental inventory reveal? Take a few moments, also, to register how you *feel* about your eating. Are you making nutritious choices? Does eating bring you pleasure? Are you satisfying your hunger?

How do you know when eating has become a balanced part of your life? We asked this same question of some of our patients, and this is what they said:

- "When I don't have to think about it anymore."

- "I know I'm eating well when I feel good."

- "I know it's right when I'm neither starving or stuffed."

- "When I can be in a situation that used to trigger overeating, and I feel perfectly in control."

- "I can go into a restaurant and be happy choosing low fat and low calorie dishes and not feel deprived."

Some or all of these responses may also be true for you. But think about the question long enough to really come up with an answer that expresses your own individual truth. You can use your answers to check in with yourself once a week or so. They can help you see when you're off course and when you're right where you want to be.

MOVE MORE: Your Muscle Mass

We now know that the average person's lean body mass declines with age. Americans, as they move from young adulthood into middle age, tend to lose about 6.6 pounds of lean body mass each decade of life. After age 45, the rate of loss increases.

According to William Evans and Irwin Rosenberg in their book, *Biomarkers: The 10 Determinants of Aging You Can Control*, "Muscle, to a far greater extent than most people realize, is responsible for the vitality of your whole physiological apparatus. . . We believe that building muscle in the elderly is the key to their rejuvenation."

Here, according to Evans and Rosenberg, are some important ways that a strong, toned musculature makes contributions to your overall well-being. A high ratio of muscle to fat on the body. . .

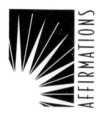

- causes the metabolism to rise, meaning you can more easily burn body fat and alter your body composition even further in favor of beneficial muscle tissue.

- increases your aerobic capacity–and the health of your whole cardiovascular system–because you have more working muscles consuming oxygen.

- triggers muscle to use more insulin, thus greatly reducing the chances you'll develop diabetes.

- helps maintain high levels of the beneficial HDL-cholesterol in your blood.

"I enjoy the healthy life I am creating."

These are good reasons to keep "moving more" right up until the very end.

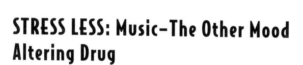

STRESS LESS: Music–The Other Mood Altering Drug

If physical exercise is like a mood altering drug, so is music. Think about your own musical experiences for a moment. Can you remember a time when you've been totally mesmerized by the sounds you were hearing and swept away into another world by a melody, a harmony, and a rhythm?

Music can both create or reflect a mood. It also has a powerful impact in helping people manage stress. Sound enters your body through your brain and can calm you down, wake you up, and stimulate your senses. If you've ever had a massage, you've probably experienced firsthand how music can also enhance a sense of deep relaxation. It is so effective as a mood enhancer that many people use music during meditation, relaxation, and visualization exercises. Music has such a powerful effect that researchers are currently exploring whether music therapy could become a way of retooling brains afflicted with a variety of emotional disorders.

Don't let yourself get so busy that you forget to enjoy the wonderful sounds available to you. Whether you're listening to Bach, the Beatles, or Anita Baker, the benefits of music are definitely there.

DAILY ACTION PLAN

Week _____   Day _____

Date _____   Weight _____

Breakfast Time:	Protein Grams	Fat Grams	Carbs Grams	Calories
Protein:				
Fruit:				
Grain:				
Beverage:				
Snack Time:				
Lunch Time:				
Protein:				
Vegetable:				
Lettuce:				
Grain:				
Fruit:				
Miscellaneous:				
Beverage:				
Snack Time:				
Dinner Time:				
Protein:				
Vegetable:				
Lettuce:				
Grain:				
Fruit:				
Miscellaneous:				
Beverage:				
Snack Time:				
TOTAL				

Today I was able to *Eat Better* by...

_____

_____

_____

_____

Today I was able to *Move More* by...

_____

_____

_____

_____

Today I was able to *Stress Less* by...

_____

_____

_____

_____

Today I feel really great about...

_____

_____

_____

_____

Tomorrow I will focus on...

_____

_____

_____

_____

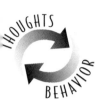

MENTAL FITNESS: Patience and Persistence

There is no way to be successful at maintenance without patience and persistence. If they're in short supply when you first start out, it's essential that you learn how to develop them as you go along.

Both patience and persistence say something important about time. Patience requires the capacity to start over again and again with confidence that you will get it right. Be conscious of not giving up too soon. Persistence requires the capacity to keep at it over time. You can see how closely they are allied.

You wouldn't be where you are today unless you had patience and persistence. Think about the time you weren't able to take effective action to change your health habits and think about the journey you have already traveled since you first began to move down this path. It may have taken you years or even decades to get to where you are now. You did it because you were patient and you were persistent. Congratulations!

DAY 54

"His work (perhaps because of the way in which I am meaning it here, the term 'vocation' is a more accurate word) provides him with a way of dedicating himself to life. Through it, or–if he is retired or if he doesn't work in the formal sense–through his hobbies and community involvements, he cultivates his talents, stands in for others, exhibits his involvement and connection to the world."
— Marsha Sinetar

Work

"Work" is a word with multiple meanings. But what if Marsha Sinetar is right when she says that your work provides you with a way of dedicating yourself to life? If we assume this statement is true, then it can be productive for you to ask yourself in what way you're dedicating yourself to life through your work.

There are very few people who can say they've spent all their working life doing work on this level. Most of us have had jobs that paid the rent for part or all of our adult lives. But even people who work at practical, rent-paying jobs can do work in the world that matters to them.

Perhaps that work involves volunteering or quilting or writing poetry or teaching a class. Work can mean something more than how you generate your paycheck.

The real question to ask yourself is whether you've found an opportunity to be productive in the world, doing something that feeds your soul, something that makes the world a better place. It's never too late, even if you have a nine to five job.

 EAT BETTER: When Eating is Only Eating

Most people who are overweight think of themselves as overeaters, at least on occasion. They are aware that there are times when they eat with a single-minded passion that doesn't admit rational thought. At such times the food they are consuming is the most important thing in their lives. They want it more than they want anything else.

You will know you have reached a balanced relationship with food when such obsessive consumption is no longer part of your life. There may still be times when you decide to go ahead and have a second helping of pecan pie, but you will be more aware of why you are doing it. You won't eat too much as a consequence of feelings or thoughts that are frightening or "unacceptable". And if you do, you'll be able to figure out what is going on.

Successful maintenance makes you stay conscious. It forces you to wake up and show up for your own life.

MOVE MORE: Second Wind

Virtually every amateur athlete experiences the phenomenon known as second wind. You probably know what we're talking about. A few minutes into your workout, you start breathing hard, your chest hurts, and your muscles burn. Then suddenly, you are pain free, energized, and flying high.

The reason this happens is that at the start of any intense physical activity, your body gets its energy anaerobically, or without using oxygen. A by-product of this process is lactic acid, which builds up in the muscles and causes cramping and labored breathing. When your body's oxygen-delivery system kicks in, you get your second wind.

Olympic athletes and other well-conditioned athletes rarely experience second wind. Their lungs and circulatory systems are efficient enough to bring lactic acid and oxygen into balance quickly, without the unpleasant effects of oxygen deficit felt by the rest of us.

Come to think of it, this is a useful analogy for maintenance. As an experienced or Olympic-level maintainer, you will be able to engage in a new activity or new way of thinking and feel comfortable maintaining it without that period of discomfort that used to come at the beginning of every new effort!

STRESS LESS: Letting A Child Choose

Today, let yourself relax into happy interaction with a child. Let a child in your life choose something he or she wants to do, and then let yourself say "Yes" to that choice.

FOOD for Thought

"If you compare yourself with others you may become vain and bitter; for there will always be greater and lesser persons than yourself."

— Desiderata

Forget the usual objections, such as "It's messy", "There isn't enough time", or "I'm too tired."

Just say "Yes". Then be there. Pay attention to how you feel during the experience. Relax and enjoy!

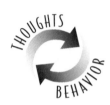

MENTAL FITNESS: More on Creativity

Today, let's take a look at more of Mihaly Csikszentmihalyi's thoughts on what ordinary people can do to experience life more creatively.

INTERNAL TRAITS.

- Develop what you lack.

- Shift often from openness to closure.

- Aim for complexity.

PROBLEM FINDING.

- Find a way to express what moves you.

- Look at problems from as many viewpoints as possible.

- Figure out the implications of the problem.

- Implement the solution.

DIVERGENT THINKING

- Produce as many ideas as possible.

- Have as many different ideas as possible.

- Try to produce unlikely ideas.

If you take even one of these ideas to heart, it will make a difference in the quality of your life. Developing your own creativity will not only allow you to become a better problem-solver, but it will enrich your days by allowing you to cultivate your capacity for curiosity and enthusiasm.

DAILY ACTION PLAN

Week _____   Day _____

Date _____   Weight _____

Breakfast	Time:	Protein Grams	Fat Grams	Carbs Grams	Calories
Protein:					
Fruit:					
Grain:					
Beverage:					
Snack	Time:				
Lunch	Time:				
Protein:					
Vegetable:					
Lettuce:					
Grain:					
Fruit:					
Miscellaneous:					
Beverage:					
Snack	Time:				
Dinner	Time:				
Protein:					
Vegetable:					
Lettuce:					
Grain:					
Fruit:					
Miscellaneous:					
Beverage:					
Snack	Time:				
TOTAL					

Today I was able to *Eat Better* by...

_____
_____
_____
_____

Today I was able to *Move More* by...

_____
_____
_____
_____

Today I was able to *Stress Less* by...

_____
_____
_____
_____

Today I feel really great about...

_____
_____
_____

Tomorrow I will focus on...

_____
_____
_____
_____

DAY 55

"No great success was ever attained alone. No one in this life ever accomplishes anything worthwhile flying completely solo, start to finish. Satisfying success is always in some way, and most times in many ways, a social product, a result of people working together. Whatever our dream is, whatever our goals are, we cannot do it alone. We did not come into this world to do it alone. We were created as social beings–beings intended to exist together and to work together in relationships. We were created to journey toward personal fulfillment with other people."

– Tom Morris

Flying Solo

It's next to impossible to do anything important and difficult totally on your own. Everyone needs someone or something to help him along the way.

You haven't gotten where you are alone. At the very least, we hope this book has been a partner for you during these past eight weeks. In the same way we hope there will come a time when you will be able to share your journey with someone who could benefit from your struggles and your insights.

You can share what it was like for you to feel unhappy with yourself and how you made the changes in your everyday habits that helped you overcome some of the obstacles. Even if you feel "unfinished" with a long way still to go, your experience will benefit someone else.

So this is a good time to thank the people who have helped you and pledge yourself to help those others who will cross your path in the future as you continue working to become your own, best self.

EAT BETTER: New Recipes

No matter how comfortable you are with your basic food routine, there's always room for something new. Eating something you haven't tasted before can be a gastronomic adventure.

One easy way to keep your eating plan fresh is to try one new recipe each week. I know people who set aside time on Sunday afternoon to plan meals for the week and to cook ahead. This is a perfect time to open that cookbook you got for your birthday last year and get creative.

Ethnic cuisine offers endless choices. You could decide today to become an expert in Chinese cooking and not come to the end of what is possible within that tradition for 30 more years.

Look for ways to keep your eating interesting to you. Try the new Thai restaurant that just opened downtown. Open your Middle East cookbook and whip up a batch of tabouli to take to work tomorrow.

MOVE MORE: One Last Plea for Keeping Track

Keeping a daily record of your physical activity will go a long way toward keeping you moving. Knowing that you're going to write it down can provide motivation when you're feeling lazy, and can grab your attention when you get distracted and start losing focus.

By now you have nearly eight weeks experience keeping track of your exercise with the Daily Action Plan. You know more about keeping track than you did before. Take this information about yourself and apply it. Find a convenient way to continue noting your activity level, and plan on doing it for the rest of your life.

Exercise is a lifeline. And since research shows that people who write down all of their physical activity actually exercise more than people who don't, keeping track of exercise clearly makes the life line even stronger.

STRESS LESS: A Simple Gift

At Lindora, we're aware of how magnificent a small, simple gift can be. We make it a practice to express our appreciation to our staff and patients as often as we can and in as many different ways as we can. When someone

DAILY ACTION PLAN

Week _____   Day _____

Date _____   Weight _____

Breakfast	Time:	Protein Grams	Fat Grams	Carbs Grams	Calories
Protein:					
Fruit:					
Grain:					
Beverage:					
Snack	Time:				
Lunch	Time:				
Protein:					
Vegetable:					
Lettuce:					
Grain:					
Fruit:					
Miscellaneous:					
Beverage:					
Snack	Time:				
Dinner	Time:				
Protein:					
Vegetable:					
Lettuce:					
Grain:					
Fruit:					
Miscellaneous:					
Beverage:					
Snack	Time:				
TOTAL					

Today I was able to *Eat Better* by...

_____
_____
_____
_____
_____

Today I was able to *Move More* by...

_____
_____
_____

Today I was able to *Stress Less* by...

_____
_____
_____
_____

Today I feel really great about...

_____
_____
_____
_____

Tomorrow I will focus on...

_____
_____
_____

gives you a magazine article they thought you might like to read, tickets to a concert they can't attend, or a shell they picked up on the beach, you feel touched. It makes you feel special. You know that someone is thinking about you, that you matter.

Knowing how good it feels to be on the receiving end makes it easy to do the giving. Sometimes people think their gifts need to be expensive, or elaborate, or artistically crafted. But deep down, we're all touched by simple gestures that remind us someone cares.

Ask yourself what simple gifts you can give to people around you that will strengthen your bond with them by showing you care, and then do it.

Your Turn.

Living With Gratitude

Today I live my life with an attitude of gratitude.

Today I am grateful for_____

_____

_____

_____

_____

_____

_____

_____

_____

_____

_____

DAY
56

"If you don't take care of your body, where are you going to live?"

– Marshall Stamper, M.D.

Congratulations!

You've completed eight weeks of maintenance on the Lean for Life program. By reading this book, following suggestions, and tailoring them to your own body and your own life, you've established the foundation for lifetime maintenance. You have what you need to continue to be free of extra weight for the rest of your life! You now have the tools to become a physically active person. It's now up to you to use the resources you have.

On this last day of the program, we want to help you retain a clear picture of your maintenance program by summarizing the basic concepts and principles. Here are ten successful strategies you will need to follow to achieve lifetime maintenance:

1. Maintain your support system. This is especially important during the next three months of maintenance. You can get support from family or friends, at one of our clinics, and from tapping into the Lean for Life web site at www.leanforlife.com. However you do it, be sure you stay in contact with the people who believe in you and can rejoice in the positive changes you're making.

2. Stay physically active. This must become a lifetime habit. How active you will need to be to maintain your weight is something you'll discover for yourself. Many people can maintain their weight by walking 30 minutes a day; some need to walk more. Many people can maintain their weight by averaging 10,000 steps a day; some need to walk farther. Becoming physically active is the single most important thing you can do for your health other than quitting smoking. You have many options for gentle exercise. Walking is just one of them. Renew your commitment to yourself–and to physical exercise–every single day.

3. Write it down. Keep track of your eating and your exercise for at least the next three months of your maintenance program. After that, if you feel that you and your weight have stabilized, you can relax your record keeping if necessary. But at the first sign of weight gain, start maintaining a Daily Action Plan again. This is one of the best ways to get yourself refocused on what you need to do.

4. Continue to weigh yourself every morning. Make morning weigh-ins a lifetime habit. Addressing a minor weight gain today is much easier than being "surprised" by a 20-pound increase six months from now. If you gain more than three pounds from your lean weight at any time during the first three months of your maintenance program, have only protein for lunch or dinner until you've returned to your lean weight. Once you've stabilized your weight, do a "Protein Day" any time you gain more than three pounds.

5. Continue eating three meals a day. Maintaining this important pattern helps train your body when to eat. If you want and need to snack, that's fine, but be sure to plan your snacks. Think in terms of protein, fruits, and vegetables. Some people have trouble digesting high-carbohydrate snacks and find themselves hungrier after they eat them.

6. Continue doing one Protein Day every week. This habit will help you maintain a sense of awareness and control over your eating and will also help curb your appetite. Many successful maintainers choose Monday as their Protein Day. Others have a protein drink for breakfast and lunch on Monday, and then have a sensible dinner in the evening. Either way, this helps balance any excess calories they may have eaten over the weekend and keeps them focused for the rest of the week.

7. Continue drinking at least 40 to 60 ounces of calorie-free liquid every day. This practice helps cleanse your system, curb your appetite, and reduce fluid retention. Also make a point to be conservative in your caffeine and alcohol consumption.

8. Continue taking vitamins. While you are probably eating healthier now than you ever have, vitamin and mineral supplements help ensure that your body gets everything it needs to operate at peak efficiency.

9. Continue practicing mental fitness. Your mental strength and your mental attitude are central components of success. Your goal is to cultivate a sense of yourself as lean and fit for life. The mental training suggestions in this book will help you develop a confident, resilient, and

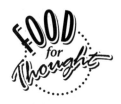

"What a wonderful life I've had! I only wish I'd realized it sooner."

— Colette

hopeful approach to life. You'll recognize problems faster and know how to solve them more effectively.

10. Continue to plan ahead for high-risk situations. You and you alone are responsible for the choices you make. You can support yourself by anticipating challenges and developing a plan of action for managing potentially difficult situations. When you know yourself well enough to know what your triggers are, and you think ahead about strategies to help you negotiate around them, you are ensuring your own success.

SUCCESS STORY: Sandra Radine

For the first time in more than 40 years, Sandra Radine's weight is no longer the focal point of her life.

"For as long as I can remember, how much I weighed–and how I looked–was something I constantly worried about," says Sandra, 60. "I started dieting back in high school. While my friends were enjoying cheeseburgers, I was nibbling 20 cherries out of a plastic bag. I never felt normal."

Losing weight was never a problem, but maintaining her weight loss success was.

"I succeeded on every diet I ever tried," says Sandra, a mother of four. "Where I failed was in keeping the weight off. One time I got down to a size 5 and bought a whole new wardrobe. Within three months, I couldn't wear any of it."

Three years ago, Sandra, who stands 5'3", weighed in at 182 pounds. She knew she had to make a major lifestyle change.

"I felt clumsy, miserable, and unattractive," she recalls. "Instead of wearing the clothes I wanted to wear, I was limited to the clothes that fit. I was also starting to feel older. I found myself thinking, 'You can't control what aging is doing to you, but you can control what you're doing to yourself.'"

Sandra committed to the Lean for Life program and lost 40 pounds. Even while battling a thyroid condition, she has maintained within ten pounds of her goal weight for three years.

DAILY ACTION PLAN

Week _____ Day _____

Date _____ Weight _____

Breakfast Time:		Protein Grams	Fat Grams	Carbs Grams	Calories
Protein:					
Fruit:					
Grain:					
Beverage:					
Snack Time:					
Lunch Time:					
Protein:					
Vegetable:					
Lettuce:					
Grain:					
Fruit:					
Miscellaneous:					
Beverage:					
Snack Time:					
Dinner Time:					
Protein:					
Vegetable:					
Lettuce:					
Grain:					
Fruit:					
Miscellaneous:					
Beverage:					
Snack Time:					
TOTAL					

Today I was able to *Eat Better* by...

_____

_____

_____

_____

Today I was able to *Move More* by...

_____

_____

_____

Today I was able to *Stress Less* by...

_____

_____

_____

_____

Today I feel really great about...

_____

_____

_____

Tomorrow I will focus on...

_____

_____

_____

_____

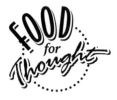

"What I value as much as the way I look is the sense of inner peace I now feel," she says. "For so many years, my weight dictated how I felt about myself. This is the first time in my life where I've truly felt at peace with my body and my appearance."

Sandra says she cherishes the sense of balance she now enjoys.

"I find that I have more time and energy to do other things now that my weight is no longer the focal point of my identity," she explains. "I still weigh myself three days a week and I maintain my food diary, but I don't obsess about it. Those things have become as much a part of my daily routine as brushing my teeth."

There used to be times when Sandra was afraid to eat because she feared regaining weight. "My problem wasn't overeating, but rather not eating enough," she says. "My doctor told me I was starving myself into obesity. I ate so little that my metabolism shut down, and everything I did eat turned to fat. These days I eat more food than I ever have, yet I still maintain my weight because I'm making healthier choices. And if I gain a couple of pounds, I no longer panic like I once did. I know what I need to do to regain control–and I do it."

YOUR FUTURE AWAITS

"Two roads diverged in a yellow wood,
And sorry I could not travel both
And be one traveler, long I stood
And looked down one as far as I could
To where it bent in the undergrowth;
Then took the other."

– Robert Frost

Over the Years

I've learned a great deal about weight maintenance from personal experience and from the experiences of thousands of Lindora patients. If I had to distill into two words the essence of what I've learned is needed for successful weight maintenance, they would be "preparation" and "faith". In order to stay the course on any path you choose, you must prepare for the success you desire. "Discovery," said Louis Pasteur, "comes to the prepared mind." Good things happen for people who are working at it. As Dr. Stamper says, you must *learn* to be Lean for Life. You must prepare to be Lean for Life.

When you do the work and then practice what you learn, you develop faith that you will be able to meet whatever challenges await you. Even if you slip up every now and then, you have faith that you will be able to get back on track. You know you have the tools, the ability to rebound, and the ability to figure things out. You can have faith in the process— and in yourself.

Danger Signs

After working with more than 200,000 patients at Lindora since 1971, we know that when people stop weighing themselves, stop keeping food diaries, stop planning meals, stop paying attention to physical activity, and stop actively engaging in mental training, they start regaining weight. We know that it's easy to slip back into old habits.

Whenever you see any of the "danger signs"—and trust me that you will—you can reach for this book, open it to any page and find that your guide, who has been with you every day for the past eight weeks, will be there for you again and again.

Good luck! May you stay healthy and may you stay Lean for Life.

"HOW MUCH CAN I EAT?"

WOMEN

ACTIVE (6,000 steps or more per day on pedometer)
12-14 calories per pound of body weight

Weight	Calories per day	Carbohydrates - 45% 1 gram = 4 cal Calories (grams)	Protein - 25% 1 gram = 4 cal Calories (grams)	Fat - 30% or less 1 gram = 9 cal Calories (grams)
100 lb.	1,200-1,400	540-630 (135-158)	300-350 (75-88)	360-420 (40-47)
120 lb.	1,440-1,680	648-756 (162-189)	360-420 (90-105)	432-504 (48-56)
140 lb.	1,680-1,960	756-882 (189-221)	420-490 (105-123)	504-588 (56-65)
160 lb.	1,920-2,240	864-1,008 (216-252)	480-560 (120-140)	576-672 (64-75)

INACTIVE (5,000 steps or less per day on pedometer)
10-12 calories per pound of body weight

Weight	Calories per day	Carbohydrates - 45% 1 gram = 4 cal Calories (grams)	Protein - 25% 1 gram = 4 cal Calories (grams)	Fat - 30% or less 1 gram = 9 cal Calories (grams)
100 lb.	1,000-1,200	450-540 (113-135)	250-300 (63-75)	300-360 (33-40)
120 lb.	1,200-1,440	540-648 (135-162)	300-360 (75-90)	360-432 (40-48)
140 lb.	1,400-1,680	630-756 (158-189)	350-420 (88-105)	420-504 (47-56)
160 lb.	1,600-1,920	720-864 (180-216)	400-480 (100-120)	480-576 (53-64)

MEN

ACTIVE (6,000 steps or more per day on pedometer)
14-16 calories per pound of body weight

Weight	Calories per day	Carbohydrates - 45% 1 gram = 4 cal Calories (grams)	Protein - 25% 1 gram = 4 cal Calories (grams)	Fat - 30% or less 1 gram = 9 cal Calories (grams)
150 lb.	2,100-2,400	945-1,080 (236-270)	525-600 (131-150)	630-720 (70-80)
170 lb.	2,380-2,720	1,071-1,224 (268-306)	595-680 (149-170)	714-816 (79-91)
190 lb.	2,660-3,040	1,197-1,368 (299-342)	665-760 (166-190)	798-912 (89-101)
210 lb.	2,940-3,360	1,323-1,512 (331-378)	735-840 (184-210)	882-1,008 (98-112)

INACTIVE (5,000 steps or less per day on pedometer)
12-14 calories per pound of body weight

Weight	Calories per day	Carbohydrates - 45% 1 gram = 4 cal Calories (grams)	Protein - 25% 1 gram = 4 cal Calories (grams)	Fat - 30% or less 1 gram = 9 cal Calories (grams)
150 lb.	1,800-2,100	810-945 (203-236)	450-525 (113-131)	540-630 (60-70)
170 lb.	2,040-2,380	918-1,071 (230-268)	510-595 (128-149)	612-714 (68-79)
190 lb.	2,280-2,660	1,026-1,197 (257-299)	570-665 (143-166)	684-798 (76-89)
210 lb.	2,520-2,940	1,134-1,323 (284-331)	630-735 (158-184)	756-882 (84-98)

WALKING OFF CALORIES

Find your current weight in the left column. The columns to the right itemize the number of calories burned based on the number of minutes walked.

Current Weight	Minutes Walked							Current Weight	Minutes Walked						
	5	10	15	20	30	45	60		5	10	15	20	30	45	60
110	20	39	61	79	114	166	225	215	36	72	108	144	216	324	432
115	20	40	63	82	118	169	234	220	37	74	111	148	222	333	444
120	20	42	65	85	123	176	245	225	38	75	113	150	225	338	450
125	21	43	66	87	127	185	254	230	39	77	116	154	231	347	462
130	22	44	68	89	132	191	264	235	40	79	119	158	237	356	474
135	23	45	69	92	136	201	274	240	40	80	120	160	240	360	480
140	24	47	71	94	141	212	282	245	41	82	123	164	246	369	492
145	24	49	74	98	147	221	294	250	42	84	126	168	252	378	504
150	25	50	75	100	150	225	300	255	43	85	128	170	255	383	510
155	26	52	78	104	156	234	312	260	44	87	131	174	261	392	522
160	27	54	81	108	162	243	324	265	45	89	134	178	267	401	532
165	28	55	83	110	165	248	330	270	45	90	135	180	270	405	540
170	29	57	86	114	171	257	342	275	46	92	138	184	276	414	552
175	30	59	89	118	177	266	354	280	47	94	141	188	282	423	564
180	30	60	90	120	180	270	360	285	48	95	143	190	285	428	571
185	31	62	93	124	186	279	372	290	49	97	146	194	291	437	582
190	32	64	96	128	192	288	384	295	50	99	149	198	297	446	594
195	33	65	98	130	195	293	390	300	50	100	150	200	300	450	600
200	34	67	101	134	201	302	402	305	51	101	155	205	305	460	612
205	35	69	104	138	207	311	414	310	52	103	157	207	310	467	623
210	35	70	105	140	210	315	420	315	53	105	158	210	315	475	631

Calculations based on walking three miles per hour and are rounded to the nearest whole number.

Lean for Life®

RESOURCES

SERVICES

ORIGINAL MEDICALLY SUPERVISED PROGRAM

The Lindora clinic system is the largest medical organization in the United States specializing in the treatment of obesity and overweight. For information on the Lean for Life clinical program, to book a free consultation, or to learn the address of a clinic near you, call 1-888-LINDORA.

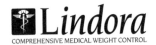

Enjoy the benefits of a weight control program in the convenience of your workplace. Health care providers such as HealthNet, Blue Cross of California, and UNICARE offer special discounts on Lean for Life programs and products. For more information regarding the "at Work" program, have your human resources or corporate wellness professional call 1-888-LINDORA.

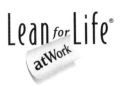

LEAN FOR LIFE at HOME At Home But Not Alone™

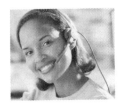

Telecoaching

If you have a telephone, you have the basic tool needed to lose weight and learn to keep it off. The At Home But Not Alone™ program combines the clinically tested weight loss program with a personal coach to guide, support, and inform you. For more information call **1-888-LINDORA.**

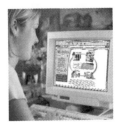

Internet

Visit our web site at **www.leanforlife.com** 24 hours a day, 7 days a week, and access the latest information on weight management, learn all about Lindora and the Lean for Life programs, e-mail your questions to our experts, participate in forums, order products and chat with others who, like you, are learning to be lean for life.

Lean *for* Life® *Online*

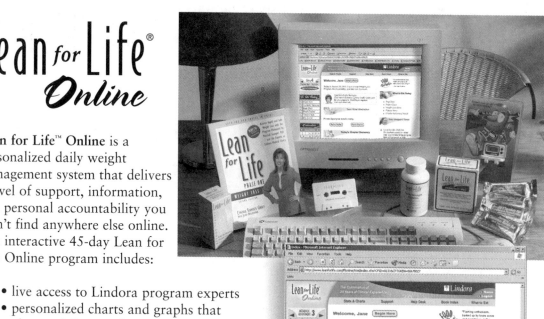

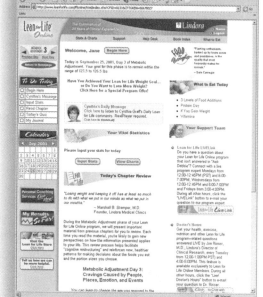

Lean for Life™ Online is a personalized daily weight management system that delivers a level of support, information, and personal accountability you won't find anywhere else online. The interactive 45-day Lean for Life Online program includes:

- live access to Lindora program experts
- personalized charts and graphs that change daily to reflect your progress
- a convenient "To Do Today" list to guide you through your program
- daily audio and e-mail messages to help keep you focused and motivated
- unlimited access to our exclusive WebPal support system
- "Ask Debbie," "Motivation Central," and expert answers to questions
- special discounts on Lindora products
- a "StartSmart" kit featuring a copy of *Lean for Life Phase One: Weight Loss* and a variety pack of delicious Lean for Life high-protein nutrition bars, a Lean for Life Activity Monitor, Fat Burning Indicators (ketone sticks), and a "Getting Started" audio tape

For more information on Lean for Life Online, go to **www.leanforlife.com** or call **1-888-LINDORA**.

PRODUCTS

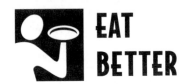

EAT
BETTER

⚕ *Lindora*

HIGH PROTEIN NUTRITION PRODUCTS

Bars • Soups • Shakes • Puddings • Drinks • Entrées

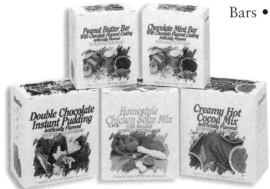

- Clinically proven to enhance weight loss and weight maintenance

- High in bio-available protein

- Low in carbohydrates

- Specifically formulated to help control cravings and maintain weight

- Convenient and Delicious

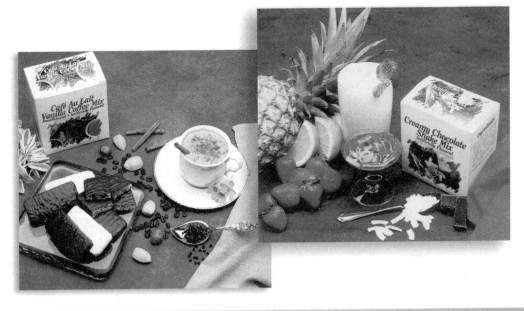

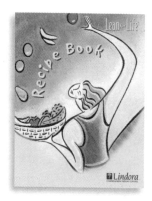

RECIPE BOOK

Recipes for everyday and for special occasions, the Lean for Life recipe book is filled with simple, delicious recipes, including many featuring delicious Lean for Life products.

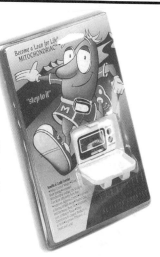

VITAMINS

These high-quality nutritional supplements are packed with vitamins and minerals and are specially formulated to enhance the Lean for Life program.

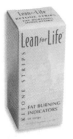

KETONE STRIPS

With these Fat Burning Indicators, you'll know immediately if you're burning fat! (For use during weight loss programs.)

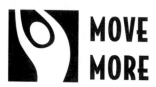

MOVE MORE

STEP COUNTER

The Lean for Life Pedometer is light, attractive, and fun to wear. A great way to be sure that you're getting the exercise you need and the results you want.

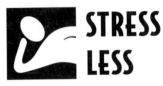

STRESS LESS

AUDIO TAPES

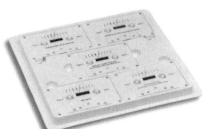

LEAN FOR LIFE Tape Series

This set of five informative, motivational audio cassette tapes includes "Getting Started: The Six Essentials," "Identifying and Eliminating Defensive Barriers," "Relaxation and Guided Visualization," "Affirmations," and "Compulsive Cravings."

MENTORS™ Daily Mental Training Audio Cassette Tapes

Herman M. Frankel, M.D. and Jean Staeheli of Portland Health Institute

As nationally prominent experts in the field of mental training, Herman M. Frankel, M.D. and Jean Staeheli work together conducting clinical programs and research at Portland Health Institute. Their tapes are designed to support you in making positive structural changes in your body and your brain.

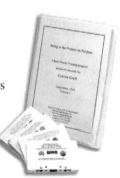

Basic MENTORS™ Program

1. My Peaceful Place
2. Enjoying My Food Choices
3. Enjoying my Physical Activity
4. Returning To The Path

Advanced MENTORS™ Program

5. Letting Go of What I No Longer Need
6. The Keeper of the Garden of Roses
7. The Child in the Chamber in the Castle
8. The Traveler and the Journey
9. My Healing Place

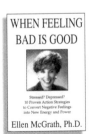

WHEN FEELING BAD IS GOOD: The Action Strategies

Spend an hour with Dr. Ellen McGrath

In this empowering 60-minute audio cassette tape, Dr. McGrath shares with you the best of what she has learned during her 28-year practice as a clinical psychologist. ACTION—not just talking and thinking—is the critical step in successfully maintaining weight loss.

BOOKS

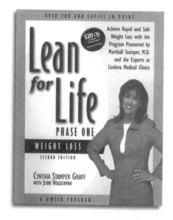

LEAN FOR LIFE PHASE ONE: WEIGHT LOSS

by Cynthia Stamper Graff
with Jerry Holderman

Lean for Life Phase One: Weight Loss is more than a book you read. It's a book you do! Whether you choose to lose five, 50, or 500 pounds, you'll find this remarkable, results-oriented book—and the clinically proven program it features—a dynamic roadmap to results. This innovative two-phase approach to weight loss has changed the lives and bodies of more than 200,000 men, women, and teens since 1971. It guides you through the program day by day, offering practical, proven "success strategies" and sharing inspiring insights from people who have lost between 20 and 450 pounds —and kept it off!

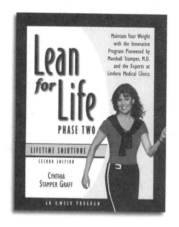

LEAN FOR LIFE PHASE TWO: LIFETIME SOLUTIONS

by Cynthia Stamper Graff

You've lost the weight. How will you keep it off? Maintain your weight with the innovative program pioneered by Marshall Stamper, M.D. and the experts at Lindora Medical Clinics. Based on more than 30 years experience, this book guides you day-by-day through an innovative eight-week program created to help you achieve a state of metabolic equilibrium. Enjoy improved health and enhanced self-esteem as you learn to Eat Better, Move More, and Stress Less.

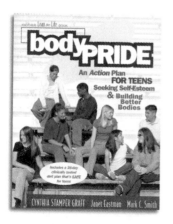

bodyPRIDE

by Cynthia Stamper Graff
with Janet Eastman & Mark C. Smith

Being a teenager can be tough, especially when you're feeling different or alone. *bodyPride* offers a motivational action plan for teens seeking self-esteem and building better bodies. This book features a 28-day clinically-tested diet plan that's safe and easy for teens. *bodyPride* is an interactive plan that supports young people in going for what they want and feeling better about what they have.

ABOUT THE AUTHOR

Cynthia Stamper Graff is president and CEO of Lindora, Inc., which manages one of the largest medical weight control programs in the United States. A nationally recognized expert in the field of weight management, she has been actively involved in the growth and development of Lindora since 1988. Graff, a leader in integrating technology into the treatment of obesity, has been instrumental in developing Lindora's atHome, atWork and online versions of the Lean for Life program. For three consecutive years, Lindora has been ranked one of the "Top 500 Women Owned Businesses in America" by *Working Woman* magazine.

Graff is the author of *Lean for Life Phase One: Weight Loss* (with Jerry Holderman), *Lean for Life Phase Two: Lifetime Solutions*, and *bodyPRIDE* (with Janet Eastman and Marc C. Smith). She is also the founder of the Lean for Life Foundation, a nonprofit organization that promotes obesity research and educational programs, and funds weight control services to selected low-income, morbidly obese men, women, and children.

An *Orange County Business Journal Women In Business* award winner, Graff is a national Ernst and Young Entrepreneur of the Year Award nominee. She has been a member of the Young Presidents Organization since 1993 and a member of Adaptive Business Leaders since 1998.

Graff holds a law degree from York University in Toronto. She resides in Newport Beach, California.